King of the Forest

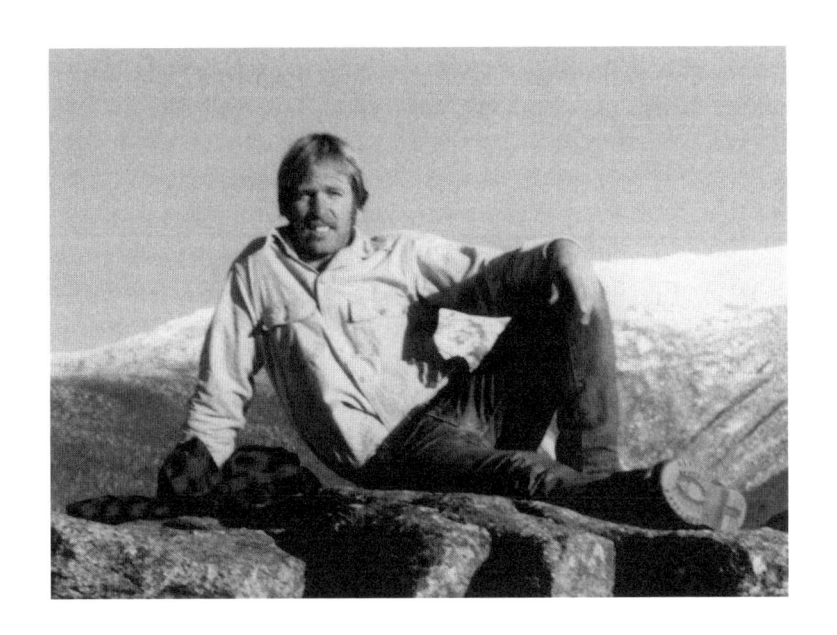

By

Lucinda Marcoux

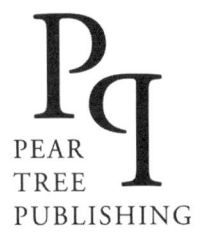

PEAR TREE PUBLISHING

King of the Forest

By Lucinda Marcoux
Copyright © 2009 by Lucinda Marcoux

Published by Pear Tree Publishing, Bradford, MA
www.PearTreePublishing.net

No part of this book may be reproduced in any form or by electronic or mechanical means including information storage and retrieval systems without permission in writing from the author, except in the case of brief quotations used in reviews. The views and opinions of the author do not necessarily reflect those of the hospitals, doctors or any other parties mentioned in this book.

First Edition

Printed in the United States of America
By Signature Book Printing, Inc. Gaithersburg, MD

Marcoux, Lucinda
    King of the Forest / by Lucinda Marcoux – 1st Ed.

    ISBN 978-0-9821983-0-8
    Library of Congress Control Number: 2008941217

    1. Title – Author 2. Family Saga 3. Health – Cancer
    I. Title II. Memoir – Lucinda Marcoux III. Biography – Ted Clark

Cover & Book Design by Lucinda Marcoux & Chris Obert
Cover Photo by Patrick Marcoux Copyright © 2009
Photo of Ted Clark by Brenda Clark Copyright © 2009
This book is printed on 60# Casablanca smooth, white, recycled paper.

Dedication

To Dad and Mom
Their unconditional love made this story possible.

Acknowledgements

I wish to thank my husband Patrick for his ever present love, respect and support through the writing, rewriting, rewriting and rewriting of *King of the Forest*. He has always been my number one fan and continues to give me the encouragement I need when I need it most. Although my daughter is a basketball player by nature, she became my personal cheerleader and for this I am forever grateful. And, I thank my son for the person he is and because I know he is there for me.

More than anything, I thank all my family and all my friends—their support and words of wisdom have given me the necessary momentum to bring *King of the Forest* to life. To my beloved family and friends I thank you a million times over!

I also wish to give special thanks to my sister-in-law Brenda who provided me with much needed medical material and factual information as well as personal insights into the day to day experience of coping with Ted's illness. Very importantly, special thanks to my mom whose diary proved to be invaluable in describing and dating the events that took place during this family story. Without the help of Brenda and Mom, I could not have put all the pieces together.

・・・

This book has been published with donations from Wheelabrator Technologies in memory of Ted Clark, former Director Environmental, Health and Safety Manager at Wheelabrator Concord and Wheelabrator Claremont.

Table of Contents

Time	7
Saddling Up	22
Talk	34
Complications	41
Into the Woods	50
Nothing Can Stop It	66
Yours is not to Question Why…	
Yours is just to Do or Die	82
Home at Last	96
King of the Forest	111
Thanksgiving	126
Christmas	134
MGH	150
The Show on the Road	165
Five Million CD 34 Stem Cells	179
Day is Done	200

Time

Ted, forty-eight years old, thinning blond/brown hair, one hundred seventy-eight pounds, and five-feet ten inches tall, gripped his kitchen telephone and pried his diagnosis out of his family physician. Ted was home alone. A short man with graying temples, Dr. Crey was miles away in his office at the hospital, but he was about to feel "the squeeze." When Ted couldn't use words he used his muscles. (As teenagers, a disgusting glance, a raised eyebrow, and hands jammed into his pockets told me it was time to back off.) If there was a way to exhibit force over the phone, Ted would find it. When he wanted me to do something I didn't want to do, he held me in a half nelson and made me shout, "Uncle."

Now, he held Dr. Crey in a similar position. Ted twisted Dr. Crey's arm behind his back and put that last bit of pressure on his pointed elbow—forcing his doctor's fingers up toward his own neck. I know it hurt.

"Tell me, or I'm leaving in the morning for my vacation." This time, Ted was not fooling around.

"No, I would like you to come with your wife and meet me in the morning at my office. This shouldn't be discussed over the phone." Dr. Crey tried to fight back.

The doctor, like me, was not as strong as Ted. We were both outmatched. Dr. Crey made a futile attempt at being released. Yet, he should have known that Ted would not let go until he got what he wanted.

Ted lowered his voice, "I'd like to know now."

I hoped my arm wouldn't break before I cried, "Uncle." Dr. Crey hoped he was doing the right thing when he gave in and said, "Ted, we think you have cancer."

It was August 7, 2002. I remember the date because it was our sister Debbie's birthday.

"Brenda, please... go to Maine," Ted told his wife. "I'll join you as soon as I get the results." It was summer and they had planned their typical outdoor, active vacation. Brenda went ahead, as she had been implored to do. Only, Ted was not going to be able to join her—his doctor's phone call put an end to that. Miles away, Brenda was finishing up her afternoon run as Ted prepared to make two life-changing phone calls. He first had to call her, and then, his dad and mom.

Ted must have been trembling in his kitchen, nervously fidgeting, knowing he must share his dreaded news. He hung up the phone and perhaps he let his guard down. Perhaps he cried uncontrollably. Perhaps he just sat. I will never know. Maybe he took a deep breath and patted his dog Jesse, a golden retriever with long, tan hair, before dialing the familiar number. How stressful this call must have been. He had to call his wife. That was difficult enough, but why did he call his dad and mom that night? He could have waited until after his wife got home and after they had a chance to meet with his doctor. What was he thinking? This burden was too much to bear alone. Ted, who had chosen to live at least an hour away from Mom and Dad, wasn't one to pick up the phone and fill them in on the minutia of his everyday life. In fact, he rarely called any of us about anything—good or bad. Nothing, prior to this message, was ever that important. Ted was less than a great communicator.

Ted's voice collapsed, crying when he called Mom and Dad. Choking he could barely get out the words, "I have cancer." Those three words infected Mom and Dad. Then, it spread to my younger brother Jim, and to me. Mom, Dad, Jim, and I live in East Kingston, New Hampshire. After Ted's call we contracted our own symptoms—extreme nervousness, fear of the unknown, and anxiety. It was a full-blown case of cancer by association. Ted was given the diagnosis of cancer, not us. Yet, we were his brother, his sister, and his parents; it was about to change us as well. In the coming months, sometimes we could only act as outside observers, other times as involved participants. Like Pac Man, Ted's errant cancer cells wanted to gobble up every good cell in his body as fast as possible and get to the end of the game. The throttle had been pushed to the start position—Ted's inner Pac Man had been released. Now, it was a matter of time.

Jim and I met in my parents' kitchen with blue and white linoleum covered flooring and blue and red rooster patterned curtains. I glanced from a cocky, colored rooster, to my mother's face overflowing with worry—(she is known to be a worrier) to a blue line in the linoleum. Then I glanced to my father's face filled with expectant tears, and back once more to a blue line in the linoleum. We were distressed. I caressed the back of one of the four wooden chairs set at the maple stained, wooden table, knowing that Mom and Dad would not be having supper there that night. Everything was put on hold as we attempted to decode Ted's diagnosis.

"How did he get it?" Jim asked, not wanting to believe the news. He was thinking about one of their dirt bike riding days.

I watched Ted and Jim tap dance across Dad's tarred driveway in their semi-professional biking shoes. Ted blinked at me as I made fun of Jim's elaborate water bottle contraption with a tube running from a "camel pack" on his back up to his shoulder. "Jim, you look like some kind of weird Martian from outer space." The colorless antenna intrigued me. "Have fun, you guys…" I watched with sister envy as the boys mounted their bikes, their bulging calf muscles pushed down on the black pedals, and I wished I was going with them. As in *The Hobbit*, the magical book that Teddy and I loved to quote, they were headed on an adventure. *The greatest adventure is what lies ahead.*

"What were his symptoms?" Jim continued to ask the questions.

Trailing in back, Jim observed the funny stroke of the pedal that made Ted wobble from side to side and tug at his pants until the crack of his butt became visible—just another thing he could poke fun of. It was a view he got from behind. From East Kingston to Kingston the roads were smooth and in twenty minutes they rounded the corner at the fire station and headed up Rockrimmon Road—the road that led to the fire tower. Toward the end where the road was paved, it became steeper and steeper until it leveled off and one by one each house was left in the distance. The huge boulder on the right side of the road marked the beginning of the dirt road. Side by side, their tires spun from black surface and onto dry dirt.

"Don't lose your pants," Jim yelled over his shoulder as he pulled ahead and cut in front of Ted.

"You asshole," Ted yelled back tightening his grip on his handle bars, bearing down even harder with his left leg.

"Owww!" Jim hollered as a heavy branch whacked his helmet and threw him off kilter. It was just the break Ted needed.

"Eat my dust," Ted laughed as he passed him and careened down the gully, spraying loose gravel in his wake.

Mano y mano; brother to brother, they dodged the dangling branches, sharp sticks, and granite boulders that flanked both sides of the road. The more rocks, the more ups and downs, the more obstacles, this was how a good ride was rated. And, the way to Rockrimmon Tower had all of this.

Streaks of blood formed jagged lines on their bare arms and legs as they scrambled to get to the tower. Ted, acting as Mufasa, and Jim, acting as Simba, were fearless, playful mountain lions. They hopped over one rock after another, and up the smooth surface of the last giant, gray boulder between them and the peak. Jimmy skidded to a stop, let his bike drop, and Teddy copied him. They reached Pride Rock—the top of Rockrimmon. It was a surface of all shapes and sizes of rocks, roots that could flip you to the ground, and moss-covered debris.

Ted's blond hair and Jim's brown hair stuck to the sides of their temples. Hearts beating hard, they slowed the pace and walked to the edge, where one false move would send them down, down, down through a thicket of brush. I thought about this, the many times I stood there, and wondered where I might end up if I tripped. It would hurt, no matter how far you fell or where you landed.

A single structure, the fire tower, reached toward the sky to an impressive height. The "look-out" was glassed-in on all four sides. Ted took off in the direction of the tower, kicking branches out of his path, noting small patches of shiny mica shimmering atop pieces of New Hampshire granite. He tugged at his biking gloves that he didn't bother to take off. In silence, Jim followed him, and the two brothers strode over to the four metal legs, ducked under the first platform, and climbed the chipped, wooden steps. Arms outstretched, Teddy teasingly grabbed the metal railings and shook them, giving Jimmy a jolt behind him. Jimmy laughed, and pulled the hair on the back of Teddy's thighs making him stumble on his loosened shoelace. "You'll pay for that," Teddy grinned over his shoulder as he continued up the long flight of stairs, stopping at the last platform. He pushed up on the trap door to the lookout, but it was locked. There was no inspector on duty, so they had the view to themselves.

Reaching the top—of anything—is reaching the top. Whether it's the top of Mount Washington, where Teddy was known to ski the headwall of Tuckerman's ravine or the top of Rockrimmon, it deserves at least a moment of reflection. Not that these two were prone to reflection, but I could envision them pausing. Teddy and Jimmy surveyed the horizon. They started far to the left, searched the middle over the tree tops, and rested far to the right. It took but a minute to cover the landscape. In sixty seconds they saw a vast sprinkling of springtime hues—the deep green of spiked pine trees, the lighter lime-like green of maples, and other grassy greens spreading across the hundred or more acres. Ted didn't miss a thing.

"There's Kingston Lake over there." Ted knew his territory.

"Yeah, but where's Greenwood?" Jim wasn't quite sure.

"Over there, behind that clearing." Ted pointed it out.

The sensual blue sky was dotted with fluffy, white clouds. Scattered streams were visible where the sun shone brightest. Ted shook his head and made a final comment before heading home.

"Man, some people have to drive hours to get this kind of view."

"How long has he been sick?" Jim needed answers.

Jimmy braced for one of his favorite parts of the road—a huge, solid obstacle buried deep in the dirt—he crouched over his handlebars. He grit his teeth as his helmet tipped down his forehead and touched the top of his eyebrows. Pedaling harder and harder Jimmy's biceps began to bulge. His cheeks, flushed red with adrenalin, were a good sign. He was determined. Rocks crunched under his tires, and tree branches whizzed by. Sure enough, he was going to face this obstacle head on. As an expert skier hits a mogul with calculated precision, aware of the course, Jimmy attacked the rock. His front tire hit the unforgiving, gray formation. Jimmy squeezed the padded tips of his handlebars even tighter. He let the law of physics take over as he and his bike careened up and over the surface. His rear tire bounced successfully on the ground—he grinned like an adolescent fully mastered at the art of doing a wheelie. In a sweeping motion he twisted his upper body backward in time to watch his older brother.

Ted roared, "Whoaaaaaaaa!!!" His arms, legs, and torso flew everywhere as his front tire pounded the rock and sent him up, and then straight back. In a flash, Ted landed on the ground with the front half of his bike on top of him. One handlebar jabbed him in the chin and his front tire pinned his shoulder. He struggled to get out from under this pile of metal as Jimmy got off his bike and strode over to inspect the damage. Jimmy saw that nothing appeared to be broken, and he collapsed, grabbing his knees. He burst into tears—laughing so hard he could hardly get out his words, "Are you all right?"

Teddy managed to get up and brush his pants off—laughing right along with Jimmy, "Yeah, I'm all right but my friggin' seat broke off." As if it was a prized dead fish, he held it up by the pointed end of the seat.

"Why didn't he know sooner?" Jim had so many questions. He knew Ted hadn't been feeling well and told him he needed to get to the bottom of it. Jim suspected something was wrong, but not cancer. What he did know was that Ted was his older brother, that he was in great physical condition, that he never smoked, that he ate well, that he was strong, and that Ted was invincible. Everything Jim knew about cancer made him feel that cures were quite possible. He'd read Lance Armstrong's book. In his confident manner Jim said, "Ted can beat this thing…I know he can."

We were a cavalry of family members being called to arms. We were summoned to guard against pending danger and we formed a posse. We had one mission. We had to get to Ted. Although we had no experience with family members getting cancer, it was instinctive to act as a troupe. We checked our cell phones, our tanks of gas, and the clock. We had time to get to Loudon before dark. We had time to figure this all out. We would make time to talk to him. My supper was planned but quickly forgotten. It was the beginning of not knowing what was going to happen, and we wanted to make each moment with Ted count. I was thinking, "What if he dies?" but never said the words out loud. As soon as the words, "Ted has cancer" registered in my brain, I began to visualize what my life would be like without him.

Why did I think this way? I'd like to think I'm not a gloom and doom person, but I had experience with death. Abigail, a friend I'd been in a dance class with, had died of breast cancer the year before. She was forty-eight. I thought of her signature t-shirt, artistically designed, with red lips on soft cotton that formed the words, "Cancer sucks." She was laughing when she pointed it out to me. Friends and neighbors bought the shirts to raise money at the June Relay for Life. We wore them with shit-eatin' grins as we circled the dirt track. I took pictures of Abigail holding the Relay for Life banner, along with other jubilant cancer survivors, as they led the first lap of the event. I nudged people aside to get a picture of her radiant smile as her husband handed her a red rose at the curve in the course.

Two months later, August 2001, the five dancing buddies met at Sal & Anthony's for supper. Abigail was having trouble breathing and was going in for surgery the next day. I called her on a whim to see if she could get together with the four of us for our periodic gathering.

"Want to meet Wednesday for supper with the rest of the group?" I was calling on a Sunday night and it was a last minute suggestion.

"Sure, that would be great. I have to have my lungs operated on the next day, but I don't have anything planned for Wednesday night. My lungs keep filling up with fluid and my doctor recommended this surgery."

"Abigail." I paused. "You're going for surgery the next day and you want to go out with us the night before? Don't you think you will want to rest and be with your family?"

"No. It will be real nice to get together. I haven't seen all of you in a while. I'll be fine."

Our five familiar faces huddled around the linen clothed table. We were cramped in a closed space that made our closeness even closer. It felt good. We told funny stories of dance recital days gone by, bragged about our children's milestones, and updated each other on important events in our lives. There wasn't a moment of silence. Abigail was thrilled when I handed her copies of the pictures from the Relay for Life. Everyone leaned over to get a good view. I knew the photos meant a lot to her.

As we parted that evening, I remember Abigail had to stop after taking four steps up the narrow, black, wrought iron steps. The stairway was tall, and steep, but it wasn't that tall.

"Are you okay?" I knew she wasn't.

She paused to catch her breath, "I just need to take my time." Abigail was determined not to make a big deal of it.

Three months later, I saw the red light flashing on my answering machine and pushed the button. Chris had left a solemn message, "Abigail is in a coma and all her family has been called. I'll let you know when I hear anything more. Chris."

The next time I saw Abigail's "Cancer sucks" t-shirt was in the photo at her memorial service. Now there were four of us.

This was not the first time I had had this kind of experience. Working for the American Cancer Society, I was all too familiar with Relays for Life. One year, a strong, determined young man with a newborn son carried the banner. He had his picture taken for the flyers announcing the event. His battle with cancer was written about in newspapers. The next year, he was gone.

These two high-spirited, athletic, goal-oriented individuals were special. I thought if someone could wish themselves to wellness,

Abigail was one that could do it. She never let on to her four dancing buddies how very sick she was. She shared her flare for the arts with a cancer support group, joking from one meeting to the next. During the two years from diagnosis to death, Abigail fought and she fought hard—but she could not beat her disease. Ted was special, but no more and no less so than these two and so many others who had died before them. Had they passed before their time or was it just their time? Could Ted beat the odds stacked so heavily against him? (He was diagnosed at stage four.)

It was early evening and there was plenty of daylight for the drive north. Summer still air surrounded our bodies as Dad, Mom, Jim, and I passed from our homes and into our cars. Ignitions in gear, Jim drove Dad, and I drove Mom. We decided to take an extra vehicle in case Ted wanted Mom to stay over for the night. It was a little decision that took a lot of thought. Would Ted want her to stay overnight? When was the last time he had called his mother for help?

Mom and I talked about this. Injuries, more than illness, were what prompted his need for her—like the time he got stung by a swarm of bees when he was about eleven years old. Ted and I were running down a hill covered with stocks of high green grass, yellow hay, and purple loosestrife. The sun was beating down on his boyish tan chest exposed to the elements. As always, he was in front, running out of my reach and I was trying to catch up. "Wait for me." I yelled, just as he began to scream. He started flapping his arms up and down, like a rooster being attacked by a stalking cat, while wild geese flew from the nearby pond. I could see a black mist swelling up from the hole in the ground and it surrounded his body. This black mist followed him in the shape of a cyclone as he tried to break free.

By the time he did, small, red blotches were springing up everywhere from his neck to his toes. Mom ran for a cold cloth, tore his pants off, and searched his skin for signs of swelling. He had been stung so many times they were hard to count. Eventually, she managed to get him calmed down. Mom didn't realize how traumatized Ted was until he required a routine shot a few months later. The doctor made the mistake of saying, "This won't hurt much…it's just like a little bee sting." That was enough to send Teddy howling before the doctor even drew up the needle.

Should Mom, or me for that matter, pack an overnight bag just in case? The last time I remembered Ted calling me because he needed something was when he was in college. He called me from a diner.

"Hey, CC, whacha doin'?" He tried to sound nonchalant.

"Nothin' much. Why?" It was unusual for him to be calling out of the blue.

"Could you come pick me up at this diner on Route 125?" He sounded lonely and far away.

"Why do you need me to do that?" I was puzzled.

"Well, I started hitchhiking home and I got this far." That was all he would say.

I hadn't had my license that long and wasn't real comfortable driving at night to places that I wasn't one hundred percent sure of where I was going. The urgency in Ted's voice overruled my fear.

"I'll wait for you by the side entrance." His words were muffled.

"I'll be there as soon as I can." I realized he really did need me.

Mom and Dad weren't around for me to ask if I could use the car. I made the decision on my own—a teenage step toward independence. I scrounged around the laundry-piled kitchen table and found the keys under a stack of newspapers. Dirt pebbles, from the unkempt carpet, blew everywhere when I started the engine; and I had to roll down the window to let some of the dust escape. (None of us, especially Ted, were very good at keeping the car clean.) The second-hand brown Chevy started on the first try, and I carefully backed it out of the driveway onto Main Street. At 9:00 at night there was little traffic on Route 125 to distract me. I kept wondering. Why didn't Ted just keep walking home or try to hitch another ride? Why did he call home? When he left Durham, he must have thought he could make it home okay. The chances of someone being at the house were fifty/fifty. As I pulled into the gravel parking area in front of the small diner, I saw Ted outside waiting for me. He looked relieved as he pushed in the scratched, silver button and opened the passenger door. Quietly, he slid in next to me.

"Thanks. I'm glad you were home when I called." He was sincere.

"Sure. No problem." I wanted to sound casual. "Did something happen?"

I was curious because it didn't seem to make sense to me. The pieces didn't fit. I hadn't known him to hitchhike and I didn't know why he decided to that night. I also didn't know what was so important that he needed to get home on that particular night. Perhaps, he simply wanted to be home. Could something have frightened him when he was hitchhiking that he didn't want to talk about? He never did.

"No, it was nothing." Enough said.

I didn't make a big deal of it, and neither did he. But, it was a bigger deal to me than I let on. I remember feeling like I had accomplished something that night that I didn't know I could. I felt proud that I could help him out. As I think about it now, this was maybe the first and maybe the last time, he had asked me to do anything for him.

Would Ted say "No," even if he really wanted Mom to stay over? He was one of her children that had chosen to live more than a phone call away, not within knocking at the door distance. Ted enjoyed his space. We knew that, but this posse of Mom, Dad, Jim, and I wanted to be prepared for the unknown—a formidable task.

Acting like good soldiers, we each took care of the crisis in front of us in the best way we knew how. It was critical for us to get to Ted, to see him, and to assess the situation. Pamphlets on *"How to Talk to Someone Who Has Cancer"* are available. I saw them every day in my American Cancer Society office. We didn't have time to read them now. Each of us would have to find our own words to express the concern we were feeling.

On the drive, I wondered would, "I'm sorry," be okay to say? Would it sound dumb or insignificant? What else could I say? Somehow it wasn't in my nature to be a cheerleader and say, "Everything's going to be okay."

Mom and I didn't speak much during the one-hour drive from East Kingston to Loudon. Memories began to flip by, like shuffling a deck of cards, one after another in no particular sequence. We had been told that one of Ted's symptoms was that he was overly tired. Lately, he'd been having trouble keeping up with his biking buddies. This was in contrast to all my memories. Physically speaking, Ted was most often in the lead.

We had a good fight over a race when I was eleven and he was thirteen.

"Cindy, I bet I can beat you from here to the mailbox and back." This was his first challenge of the day.

"I'll race you, but you have to ride the bike the long way and I'll run the short cut across The Plains." I accepted the challenge on my conditions.

Our big, old, white colonial house was smack dab in the middle of Kingston where "The Plains"—as the locals call the open, park-like squares through the center of town—are still sectioned off between the paved side roads. The side roads have little traffic and connect the two main roads that run parallel down the center of town. From our house down to the side road, across the side road, down the other road, to the mailbox and back was about one quarter of a mile. My route, a straight shot from the house, across The Plains (watch out for the big ditch) to the mailbox and back, was half of that. In my immature mind, I figured I had a good chance at beating him.

We were two racing professionals setting up in the blocks. We took our positions. Ted, with his tussled, blond hair, mounted his Sears special, "high speed" racing bike. My toes, poking through the sides of my Converse sneakers, gripped the rubber soles. I was, *aquiver with anticipation*, as I knelt over, placing left hand over right hand, on my bent right knee. It was a familiar, "brace for competition" pose. Ted started the count, "On your mark, get set, go!"

Woooshhh, every ounce of energy surged from my brain cells down to my toes and with a gust of wind I was off. So was he. I flew (short brown hair flopping up and down) across the street, jumped over the ditch, and targeted the mailbox. Never once did I dare to look to my right to see where he was. In minutes, I tagged the mailbox, circled around it, and bee-lined it back across the grassy field. I was running like my life depended on it. Ted was biking just as fast as he could. Upon reaching our yard, I caught a glimpse of him out of the corner of my eye as he dropped his bike on the ground and ran for the house. Head down and hunching my shoulders, I gave a last ditch effort.

We tripped up the porch steps and slammed into the aluminum door nearly knocking each other over, both tagging it at the same time. It was too close to call, but we tried to anyway. Resembling Jem and Scout, in *To Kill a Mockingbird*, we argued with a passion for what we thought was right.

"I won!" I jumped up and down, almost tripping over Tiger our multicolored cat.

"No, I won!" Like Jem, angry with his obnoxious little sister, he huffed and he puffed—his scrawny, tight chest pointing in my direction.

"No, sa!" I got even closer to his chest.

"No, sa!" He towered over mine.

"I won!" Like Scout furious with Jem, I kicked the step and yelled in his face.

"No you didn't!" He grabbed my wrist and began to bend it backwards. I hated that move, but it forced me to conjure up all my strength and focus on getting out of it. If I managed to make a fast enough jerk that was strong enough, he would have to let go. That was satisfying.

"You just can't admit that I won!" Screaming, I wrenched my wrist to the right and tried to snap it out of his pincer grip. It didn't work and he squeezed even tighter.

Mom could hear us from the kitchen and hustled her way to the porch. She burst through the screen door, launching her own attack. "Go to your rooms until you can come out and make up!"

She didn't have time to listen to our stories. The solution needed to be quick. We understood her words and reacted to them. Sweat soaked hair stuck to our cheeks and droplets of water dripped onto the steps. Tiger slipped between our bare legs as we stepped forward. One loose wire from the torn screen door pierced my shoulder as I pushed past Teddy. We took our dirty red faces, plastered on white skin, into the kitchen and parted without saying another word. He stomped off to his room and I stormed off to mine.

"Ted has been taking antibiotics on and off over the past several months and when he went in for these last tests, he thought he might have Lyme disease." Mom broke my train of thought.

"What made him think he had Lyme disease?" I pulled to a stop at an intersection and watched a tan SUV cross by.

"He thought some of his symptoms—like fevers, muscle aches, and headaches—might be caused by Lyme disease. He is out in the woods all the time. I guess he's been reading about it on-line." Mom was stating the facts.

"I wish he had been right." I said, and then, the ace of diamonds flashed by as I remembered my nephew's wedding back in June.

It was at this wedding that I first learned Ted had not been feeling well. Nothing specific, he just wasn't himself. Brenda said he didn't feel like staying over at the hotel, like some of us were doing. How does a doctor make a diagnosis out of someone not acting like themselves? For me, if I stopped dancing, that wouldn't be myself. My family would know something was wrong. With Ted, it was the difficulty with his bike riding and a persistent cough. We knew something was wrong.

I made my way across the flat, smooth, wedding reception-room floor. Conversation clicked around us and I eased up to Ted within talking distance. His shoulders shifted uncomfortably under the obligatory blue suit. The white shirt, a bit wrinkled, was obligatory as well. His eyes darted my way as he flashed me his receptive smile.

"Hey, CC, how you doin'?" His hands in his pockets, he rocked from one foot to the other and shifted his upper body. He had a nickname for all five of his sisters and I always chuckled when he called me CC. I guess you could call it a term of endearment.

"Great. But, I want to know about you. I hear you haven't been feelin' so good lately. What's goin' on?"

"It's no big deal. I just have this cough that won't go away. I've been feelin' kind of so-so." Ted's mouth changed, his lips shrugged. He wanted to smile but he couldn't.

He was quick to change the subject, "How's your granddaughter? She's a cutie."

"Yeah, she's pretty special." We glanced toward the floor where Ashton was twirling in her pretty blue party dress. Wisps of her straight, blond hair covered her eyes. I can always count on a child to shift my concentration from the heavy thoughts in life, to the lighter ones. Ted and I stopped talking to watch Ashton and her cousin, Jason, run between and around the dressed-up legs of the wedding guests— just like playful kittens. Head down, Ted began to drift. Was he wondering if he would ever get to see his grandchildren?

Mom and I turned the corner onto Piper Hill Road and drove toward Ted's house. Green oak and maple leaves canvassed the sky, lining each side of a somewhat familiar road. A weathered, wooden fence rail, slanted down to the ground, marked the edge of his property. That's how I knew we were close. I glanced across the pond Ted had dug, surrounded by high grass and weeds, and caught sight of his brown shingled gazebo.

Jim and I turned into the driveway and stopped in front of the garage. We opened the car doors. In slow motion, the four of us made our way across the yard, as Ted was coming up the knoll from his gazebo. Inch by inch, step by step, slowly I come. We used to play this game when we were young. He would say it softly in a tease, slightly under his breath, "inch by inch, step by step," then a little louder "inch by inch, step by step," then a little louder "inch by inch, step by step" – making my heart beat a little faster each time—until he would take off after me, and I would run away as fast as I could. This time, it was not a game and I was not going to run away.

I watched him plod up the small incline—not used to seeing him move so slowly—making my heart beat in time with his. He looked like he was carrying the eighty-pound knapsack he lugged through the snow-covered mountains in Outward Bound. Today, there was no snow-covered mountain and there was no eighty-pound knapsack. Pesky mosquitoes buzzed all around us infesting the humid air. Ted, in his light-weight cotton shirt, was carrying a heavy burden. He tried to look encouraging as he greeted us at the top of the knoll, but it didn't work. He was shaking. Dad, Mom, and Jim met him with a hug. I did too. My arms reached around his waist and he pulled me in close; neither of us wanted to make the first move to separate.

Together, we walked to the screened-in gazebo; it was another tight-knit group, in another tight-knit space. An enclosed gazebo—not altogether outside and certainly not inside—it served as a transition room. We were leaving one space and entering a new one. Ted was known as an athlete, husband, father, son, brother, and friend. It reminds me of those intellectually stimulating workshops where I have been asked, "Who are you?" I have answered, "A wife, mother, daughter, sister, friend, and dancer." All through our lives we are identified by who we are to others, and by what we do. We are asked, "How do you see yourself?" Ted could add a new description to his list—a cancer patient. What would that mean? We each took a place at the round table in the center of the gazebo.

Watching out for mosquitoes breaking through a hole in the screen, I heard Mom ask, "How are you feeling?" My mom: the nurse, the mother, the worrier, the communicator, the nurturer, had to ask.

"Not so good." Ted could hardly get out the words, his mouth having difficulty interpreting the signals being sent from his brain. His lips quivered as he looked to the floor.

As I focused on his face, searching for words, all I kept thinking was, "He is in deep trouble." His skin was bilirubin yellow. Bilirubin, a product broken down in the blood system, is an indicator that the liver is malfunctioning. The skin turns a dingy, tell-tale yellow. (Ted was born with yellowy-tinged skin—it was a distinguishing factor in his birth.) He told Mom that his bilirubin count was always high. I remembered Mom describing her big, nine-pound baby. He was the heaviest of her seven. After delivering three healthy baby girls, Ted was her first son. He was late to arrive but was strong and thriving, in spite of the abnormal bilirubin. Teddy was a big eater from the start—she had trouble keeping up nursing him.

In addition to his unhealthy skin color, Ted's cheeks were puffy; like someone on Prednisone. But he wasn't. I kept thinking, "He even looks sick." I had seen people with cancer, and some of them didn't look sick. Ted did not look good. It wasn't just his distressing skin color and puffy cheeks that made me feel this way. When Ted's vacant, blue eyes searched for answers from Dad, Mom, Jim, and me, I saw they were filled with uncertainty, and with fear.

Saddling Up

The message that Ted had cancer was delivered from one address, to another address, to another address. It went to family—in-laws, cousins, nieces, nephews, aunts, and uncles—as well as friends—from high school days from college days, from past and present work days, from biking groups, and from neighbors in the neighborhood. It was not delivered in rose-colored wrapping with a big red bow, easy to unwrap and a delight to touch and feel. It was more like a heavy, brown envelope from a lawyer, in the middle of a law suit, where a glance at the return address makes you want to faint. You go numb in the head and everything around you becomes a blur. You feel dizzy knowing that the news must not be good but you have to open it up to see for sure. You hold your breath while you break the seal. If you ignore it and don't open it, things are likely to get worse. So you do. Then, you start reading the letter and find that you have a hard time understanding the words; they are confounding to you. You discover that you have to learn a new language—legalese, just like you will have to learn medical terminology. It will take professional interpretation to be educated in the technical jargon. Ted, his family, and his friends had to begin to learn cancer terminology, a language filled with unknown codes and intimidating information.

The first translation that had to be made was the diagnosis of cancer being defined as a specific kind of cancer. This could only be done after the data was collected from a number of tests. The tests follow the symptoms. Symptoms can include: enlarged lymph nodes (usually in the neck or armpit) fever, night sweats, and weight loss. In Ted's case, he had experienced chronic colds during the spring of 2002 and been in and out of the doctor's office. He was treated for cold and sinus infections, put on antibiotics, and attempted to resume his normal routine, that included long, strenuous bike rides. While on the first course of antibiotics he appeared to get better and he took it as a good sign. But it wasn't long before he was back at the office for a second, a third, and a fourth course of antibiotics, each time becoming a little more lethargic. Still, he was thinking it was no big deal.

By May, there were times when he would wake up and his sheets would be damp; his fevers had reached high enough temperatures to push the sweat right out of him and it was only spring. How odd to wake up and find oneself in this kind of predicament—he was not a woman in midlife going through menopause, he was not his young son with a childhood virus—he was, supposedly, a healthy adult male. Ted and Brenda thought the night sweats were all part of the infection working its way out of his body so they were not alarmed. They hoped the antibiotics would take care of it.

By June, the night sweats were becoming more frequent and by July, his rumpled bed sheets were not damp—they were soaked. What an embarrassing, uncomfortable sensation to wake up in a pool of wetness.

"What the hell is this mess all about?" Ted kept asking.
"I don't know. It has to be something with your infection. I'll clean it up." Brenda went about her business and tried to make sense out of this nuisance in their lives.

At the end of July, lethargic and pale, Ted saw his family physician who thought he might have a heart infection. He ordered a CT scan and blood work just to be sure. It was no heart infection, it was cancer. After the diagnosis of cancer was made, a specialist, an oncologist, was brought into the treatment phase. More tests were taken to determine what kind of cancer Ted had. Thankfully, a surgeon at Concord Hospital found an enlarged lymph node in Ted's neck that could be biopsied. Removing tissue from his neck was less painful and less intrusive than if they took it from an enlarged node that had grown in his back.

In the world of a Maasai tribesman, a sign of bravery is "facing the lion." Elephants, rhinos, buffalos, and hyenas are merely wild animals to be dealt with. The lion—a symbol of bravery and pride—is much more than a wild animal. It takes on a revered status in the African Savanna. If a Maasai tribesman, no matter how old he is, stands his ground and kills a lion—great tribute is paid to him. Warriors sing songs about how brave they are. It is a cultural rite of passage to "face the lion." In Ted's case, within the framework of medical technology and advanced treatments for cancer, Ted would face his own rite of passage. He would need to "face the needles." And, he would need to face them over and over again.

I don't know anyone that likes needles—except for nurses, lab-technicians, and junkies, but there are those that dislike them more than others. Ted was one of those. Perhaps, it was his early indoctrination via bee stings that gave him a dislike of needles. It's one of those memories that *sticks* with you. Or, perhaps it was due to the numerous trips to the emergency room where shiny, silver, sharp points stuck him in injured places.

Two unshapely apple trees sprawled over our dirt driveway where they dropped sticks, leaves, and rotten apples under foot. Soft, squishy, bruised apple skin oozed up between the cracks in my toes—I wasn't watching the ground as I searched for a red Frisbee. A yellow blossom syringa bush beside the well was in full bloom and the handle to the rusty, push mower (Ted and I fought over who would mow the lawn) lay prone between the house and the barn. Jimmy had just jumped off the swing in front of the barn and was headed to the garden out back when the wheels of Teddy's skateboard hit the abandoned yellow Tonka truck not far enough away from the well cover. Like a dropped banana peel lying in wait for its victim, the toy Tonka truck was destined to bring someone down. It did.

The front two round, dirt-covered wheels hit the back end of the unloading dump truck and flipped Teddy up in the air and over backwards onto the cement well cover. The impact of his head against the hard surface created a small chasm from the nape of his neck to the curve in his skull. I didn't want to look and ran to get Mom. Blood seeped from the abyss and left burgundy droplets on the cement, the ground, and the grass. Bundled in blood soaked towels he was rushed to the emergency room. I waited anxiously at home.

I bit off the nail on the tip of my index finger and chewed on it as our black Corvair pulled in the driveway. Teddy climbed out of the back seat—his white, Fruit-of-the-Loom, t-shirt stained with blood and dotted with dirt.

"What did they do to you?" I asked timidly.

"Stitched me up. Wanna' see?"

Before I could answer, he turned his back to me. He gave me a full view of his partially shaved head engraved with tiny knots and black tips of taught surgical thread.

On that end-of-summer morning when Ted went for his biopsy, he was surprisingly calm—not nervous about the procedure at all.

Perhaps the relief that something, anything, was being done to make steps toward a cure for his ailments reassured him. He had already been told that he would not have general anesthesia—he could remain partially awake.

"How are you Ted?" The surgeon asked looking straight into his eyes. "You understand what we are going to do here?"

"Yup. Just do what you have to do."

As the surgeon drew up a size twenty-two needle and filled it with Novocain, he continued to ask Ted questions.

"How's the biking going?" He knew Ted was a biker.

"Not so good." Ted hadn't been feeling well enough to go on any long rides.

"Well, I hope you're able to get out there pretty soon."

"Yeah, me too."

In about eight minutes flat the surgeon had sliced through the outer layer of skin, removed the peanut-sized node, and stitched him back up.

"We'll get the report to you as soon as possible." The surgeon assured him as Ted left to meet back up with Brenda in the waiting room.

During summers, Teddy and his cousin Skippy, who was two years older, worked on "the farm" owned by our Uncle Harry. In contrast to Teddy's blond hair, Skippy's was black. And, he was a few inches taller. Skippy was a lean, athletic machine—even in his teens. It was before they could drive, so they rode their "no-speed" bikes six miles from Kingston to Kensington to earn a few bucks helping to clean the cow pens, milk the cows, and hay. To cool off during the middle of the day, they rode their bikes to the blood-sucker infested farm pond. (We always had to inspect our bodies to make sure a huge, black blood-sucker wasn't sucking the blood out of one of our legs.)

"Hey Ted, let's go swimmin'." Skippy nudged him, as he threw a shovel of shit on Ted's lower pant leg. They were surrounded in black dung glistening in the afternoon streaks of sunlight passing through the open barn windows. Black flies surrounded them too.

Teddy shrugged, swatted a fly and leaned his shovel against the edge of one of the window frames—breaking an elaborate spider web. He turned away from the calves and headed for his bike. Eager to get to the water they peddled standing up. They bobbed and weaved all the way from the barn with the milking parlor to the pond nestled at the base of hills—covered in hay fields. Rows of corn stalks could be seen in the distance.

Simultaneously, they slammed on their brakes at the foot of a humongous boulder. They dropped their bikes at the brown, wooden "changing-shack"—where cousins changed into bathing suits—and ran down the hill. With limited time, they skipped the "changing-shack," stripped down to their "whitie tighties," and threw off their shit-kickers. Bare-chested, they raced to the murky water. On his way, Teddy reached up and swatted a low-lying branch from the fast-growing weeping willow. (I remember how quickly it spread its intricate wings across the rough lawn in front of the pond.) They kept running as stiff stalks of cut grass stabbed at the bottoms of their feet. Reaching the sandy shoreline and cool water, they raised their arms over their heads, in diving position, and dove in head first. They stayed under for as long as they could hold their breaths—a form of competition. Nasty horse flies hovered over their heads waiting for them to resurface.

And, the horse flies were there to follow them out of the water and to the diving boards—one high and one low. In jungle-gym climbing fashion, Skippy climbed up the ladder of the high diving-board. He ran to the edge, bounced up and down a few times (this board had a lot of spring) and did a swan dive. At the time, they were into swan diving. Water collected on the end of the wooden diving-board. It made it slippery.

Teddy, dripping wet, came out of the water and onto the same diving-board. He also ran to the end of the diving-board and started to bounce up and down. The water on the bottom of his feet hit the pool of water on the edge of the long wooden plank and yanked his feet out from under him. His body went out of his control. Like a whirling dervish, Teddy's arms and legs flailed in the open air. His head whacked the diving-board on the way to the water below—he never saw it coming.

The hit knocked the wind out of Teddy but he was not unconscious. Skippy wrapped an arm around Teddy's chest and helped him swim back to shore. Blood left a trail in the water and across the sand as they walked to their bikes—they had to ride back to the farm. Teddy struggled to hold his t-shirt to the back of his head as he pedaled up the dirt road. He was thinking, "I know this is gonna need stitches."

The diving-board accident was the second major blow to his head and second set of major stitches. The blow on this day would be far worse.

It was a long day. The air in the waiting room became cooler and cooler as night time approached; other patients and their family members had come and gone. A yellow vinyl couch and matching chairs took up space in the magazine-filled waiting room. A floor lamp was tucked in between the chairs in the corner of the room, poised to shed a faint light. A soft-spoken nurse offered Brenda warm blankets to ease her visible chills. She gladly wrapped them around her. Ted was silent as he sifted through the pages of *Sports Illustrated*. The doctor appeared at the door, pulled up a chair, and looked from Ted to Brenda, then back to Ted.

"We think its Hodgkin's lymphoma. The good news is that Hodgkin's lymphoma is very curable." Ted and Brenda left that evening with a ray of hope that, although it was going to be a struggle, his cancer could be beaten.

They began their research—what is this thing called "Hodgkin's lymphoma?" (Thomas Hodgkin, a British physician, first identified this type of malignancy in 1832—close to one hundred and seventy years ago.) This cancer has been around for quite some time. It's a form of cancer that affects the lymphatic system. Jim and I, and the rest of us, learned that the lymphatic system is a sophisticated network of vessels and organs that transport, produce, and store lymph. Lymph is clear, watery, and sometimes a faintly yellowish fluid that comes from body tissues that contain white blood cells. It circulates throughout the lymphatic system until it returns to the venous bloodstream through the thoracic duct. It supplies mature lymphocytes to the blood, as well as removing bacteria and certain proteins from the tissues. Lymph is important to our life support system in the same way chlorophyll is to photosynthesis—without it, plants die; without it, we die. Yet, we don't think about lymph the way we do other vital parts of our bodies. We don't say, "I'd really like to get into his lymph, or he really gets under my lymph, or he really gets on my lymph." I could see what the dysfunction of the lymph system was doing to Ted's body, but I could not see what it was doing to his mind, and I wanted to get into his head.

I was haunted by the unknown. I didn't want to dissect his disease the way technically-oriented, engineering-type persons would. To examine the details has never been my thing; Meyer's Briggs tests have proven me to be a more "global thinker." I tend to look at the big picture, sum it up, make a quick assessment, and want to get to the bottom line. When people asked me specifics about Ted's illness, I didn't have the answers. I knew he was sick, I knew he would be treated, and I knew he may or may not get better. The vast amount of details like what is chemotherapy, what drugs are used in chemotherapy, how many treatments are enough, why chemo and not radiation, how do the doctors know what is best—all became a blur. I wanted to know the emotional side of what Ted was experiencing. I wondered; what was he feeling?

It was any Saturday morning in the fall of 1971 and I got up early. Even though it was a Saturday morning, I got up early. I knew I needed to do my chores before I could leave for the football game. I wanted to be able to join my cousin Kathy (Skippy's sister) and my best friend Brenda, for the walk to the high school. Kathy and Brenda were much shorter than me (we were all the same age)—each around five-feet and three inches tall. We all had long hair (it was a carry-over from the 60s) but each a different color. Kathy had straight blond hair, Brenda had thick black hair, and mine was plain brown. I had to vacuum the living room before I could "go out and play." (I knew they'd be waiting for me because they didn't have as many chores to do.) As I pushed the black triangular attachment in between the red, upholstered cushions I glanced out the front windows onto The Plains thinking about the game—I hoped no player would get hurt. My freshman year, and Ted's junior, Sanborn Regional still had football—it would be cancelled the following year due to lack of players and lack of money. The Sanborn team was small and it was tough, but it wasn't real tough.

It wasn't the smell of the germ-infested—there was an outbreak of impetigo—gym that made Ted puke his guts out before this game and every other high school football game. It was nerves. As Pat, one of his best buddies, pulled his floppy shoulder pads down over his head and looked to his right, he saw the color drain from Ted's face.

"Hey, Ted, how yeah doin'?" He nudged him as Ted searched for the wastebasket on the other side of their bench.

Under his breath, Ted mumbled, "Great," as he bent over and grabbed his stomach. He let out a bit of a gurgle and then began to hurl. Chunks of orange, yellow, blue, and red hit the gray metal and dripped down the sides of the bucket, landing in a puddle at the bottom. The smell of his own vomit smacked him in the face. Bending up straight, Ted took the back of his hand and swiped it across his mouth, cheek, and tip of his ear.

"Let's go, guys!" Coach Dawkins yelled from the door.

In the words of the immortal John Wayne—*Courage is being scared to death, but saddling up anyway.* Ted adjusted his sloppy shoulder pads under his tight, white uniform with blue letters. He was thinking and he was feeling, but he wasn't talking. He listened to Coach Dawkin's pre-game speech and kept his thoughts to himself.

Coach Dawkins ended with less than inspirational words of encouragement, "Go get em'!" Joining the line of clomping football cleats, Pat and Ted bumped chests. As they ran from the locker room to the field, a glob of orange, consumed at breakfast, clung to a strand of blond hair sticking out from under Ted's helmet. I could see it from the bleachers.

Nerve, lymph, muscle, organ, and brain cells are all interconnected. There is a connection between the mind and the body, and the body and nature. People may ignore the symptoms, but they are there. Some people get ulcers and we never see what those ulcers look like. Some people have outbreaks of psoriasis and it is there for everyone to see. Some people have anxiety attacks. If we could only interpret the warning signs before we crash. Flashing yellow lights blink, warning us to slow us down, yet we are tempted to speed up and go even faster to beat the red light. We want to speed through each passing intersection. I suffer from migraines and it took me a long time to read the signs; the yawning, the lightheadedness, the creeping in of fatigue. I would ignore these things and try to complete just one more task until my body stopped me dead in my tracks. Now, my brother was stopped dead in his tracks. Did he ignore the warning signs and keep trying to do one more task?

Ted was "sort of sick" for about two years. Symptoms too vague to make him go to the doctor prohibited him from getting a thorough work-up. Besides, why would someone as healthy and active as Ted suspect that something was drastically wrong? Coughing his way to work he went on; he bottled up any work-related stress and hoped he would get better. Stress can cause a multitude of health problems and side effects especially if it is never talked about. Can it trigger cancer cells to go wild? Would Ted have been healthier and happier working on the farm?

Ted banged the door and started into the kitchen—his sticky, dirty arms spattered with loose, yellow hay—like paint specks on a painter's overalls. His smelly dungarees (note the "dung" in dungarees) were crusted with crap from shoveling manure and milking the cows at dawn. He started to walk across the 60s, red-brick linoleum floor.

"Take your boots off and leave them on the porch!" Mom was on to him. Ted's shit-kickers should never have come in the house, but they usually made it as far as the entryway before Mom would catch him.

"Ted, how many times do I have to tell you to leave your work boots on the porch? And leave your dungarees on the bathroom floor; I don't want them in with the rest of the laundry." And…neither did I!
Ted didn't see the need for a response. He glanced at her sideways and slunk away, just like a cat ignoring its owner. His hair looked like he had just come through a wind tunnel and he really didn't care. It was his style.

"What's for supper?" He directed the question at me.

"I don't know. You'll have to ask Mom." I brushed him off.

I did feel bad for him though, and wondered how he'd made it through his day. He was suffering with an itchy case of poison ivy—something he was prone to catch in the middle of the hottest summer days. Earlier in the week, I saw a few raised spots on his hands and fingers. For his sake, I'd hoped it wouldn't break out all over. Unfortunately, it did spread to his arms and chest, and before long it was all over his cheeks. Now, his eyes and his eyelids were swollen, making it hard for him to see. Another day of this and he'd probably need a shot of Prednisone. Lines of bubbles and blistered blotches covered in Calamine lotion made him look like a pink ugly monster from *Fantasmic Features*. (We used to watch that show together.) He played up the part hovering over me, arms arched, fingers wiggling with a delirious look in his eyes poised to spread his poison. In a deep, yet squeaky voice his words drawled out, "I'll get you my pretty and your little dog Toto, too…" In spite of his wicked threat, I had to laugh.

The heat, the open spaces, the barns, and the tractors were a natural fit for Ted. Riding alone and uninterrupted around the "Bentz Field"—each of the fields has a name—in scorching temperatures was far better than cooking fried clams at "Bolton's," the local clam stand, which didn't suit him at all. Driving a tractor over miles of fields gave him plenty of hours to be lost in thought. There was no pesky boss harassing him about putting too many clams in a clam box. I wonder what he was thinking about as he plowed over rows of hay steering number eight hundred twenty-six (each tractor had a number) through wide open fields with the blazing sun on his face and a faint breeze on his back. As did Bilbo Baggins, Ted felt the love of beautiful things.

Unlike other forms of cancer, that may be localized, Hodgkin's lymphoma affects more than just one organ in one part of the body. It can spread anywhere and everywhere. Ted's cancer cells were as contagious to his body as the news of his cancer was to his family. We internalized and externalized our feelings in our own way. Jim attacked it one way. He sought answers from professionals, went on-line, read articles, and talked at length with doctors he knew. I continued to hear the information but not necessarily absorb it, wanting, as usual, to get to the bottom line. I asked myself, "In the end, will he make it or will he not?" And in the meantime, I wondered, "What is he thinking?"

Shoveling cow manure and slinging seventy-pound bales of hay was a great way for Teddy to stay in shape. To test how fit he was, we played the "grunch it" game. I made a tight fist with my right hand, held it firm near his waist, and told him to get ready.

"Grunch it," I yelled.

On command, he contracted his abdominal muscles and braced for the blow, trying not to laugh. My fist bounced off the middle of his stomach, like feet hitting a trampoline. I don't know why I got such a kick out of doing this, other than the fact that it was the only time that I could hit him without fear of being hit back. It was more evidence of something he had that I didn't, a male muscular physique. When I was little I tried to pee standing up, just because he could and I couldn't. No matter how much I exercised, my stomach would never look or feel like his. His trained, teenage muscles produced a rope-like rippling, over tanned skin envied by body builders. I thought it would be great to have muscles that tight. My puny little punch came up short every time, but the effort was empowering.

It also gave me a feeling of power to play in pick-up football games on The Plains. Teddy hollered to Skippy, Kathy and Brenda who were walking across our neighbor's yard.

"You guys gonna play?" Teddy asked.

"Yeah, we're in."

Brenda was hangin' out with Kathy and she was game. And, it didn't take us long to round up enough players from the neighborhood to pick teams. Today, Dexter Snyder came to play. He was six-foot tall and solid muscle—Paul Bunyan would've been an apt nickname—he cut down anyone in his path. (His real name was kind of funny, but nobody dared to make fun of it.) And, the Snyders had a reputation for being wild. I pretty much kept my distance. I couldn't tell you the color of his eyes, because I tried not to look at them. Teddy and Skippy—two of the toughest, most-respected Sanborn football players—called out various names and we went to one side or the other. We saw a passer-by walking up the street and Teddy waved him over to even out the numbers.

"Watch out for the ditch," I yelled to this unknown guy, who wasn't aware of the foot-deep trench.

My warning came too late. The passer-by was looking at Teddy when his knee buckled and he tumbled into the dirt. It was like watching Arte Johnson from *Laugh-In*, hunched over on an undersized bicycle, peddling as fast as he could and then suddenly tipping over on the tar. One minute he was up and the next he was down—the unexpected abruptness made me laugh. Teddy lifted his left eyebrow at me and without speaking said, "You shouldn't be laughing."

Chemotherapy was prescribed. Like everyone who has heard about cancer, I had heard about chemotherapy, been vaguely familiar with it, and knew there were possible side effects. Now, I would be forced to know the details of chemotherapy—they call it a "cocktail"—but no one would choose to serve it to a friend.

Ted's first cocktail was called ABVD, consisting of the drugs Adriamycin, Bleomycin, Velban, and Dacarbazine. Each of these drugs alone could be used to treat other diseases. Each drug came with its own set of side effects. Ted was scheduled to receive a total of twelve treatments, consisting of two times per month for six months.

"Hut one, hut two, hut three," Teddy called out, reaching under the passer-by's legs. (This was a good reason for me to shy away from playing quarterback.) A mad scramble of legs in organized confusion darted left and right while chest-to-chest contact was made. The passer-by headed for the imaginary goal line waving his hands for the ball. Teddy sent the football down-field, but Dexter reached up and intercepted the pass.

Dexter, or Paul Bunyan if you prefer, elbowed his oncoming opponents and took off in the direction of the gray sweatshirt marking one corner of his end zone. I saw him coming and took off after him. No one was paying any attention to miss little ole female me so instinctively I dove for his ankles. I wrapped both my arms around his right leg and pulled back as hard as I could. My meager young chest deflated—hitting the solid turf. And, Paul Bunyan, like an oak tree falling amongst saplings, crashed to the ground. Players witnessed the fall, but never heard a thing. At first I thought he might come after me, but instead, he got up, brushed off his pants and turned his back. No one said a word. It empowered me to take down a guy his size and stature. Without an older brother, I never would have had the balls!

"You'll probably feel okay after the chemo treatments." The nurses told Ted, but he was concerned about his "easy nausea"—which regularly set in about two days post chemo. Brenda and Ted went out to eat after his treatments, like a child being treated with ice cream after a visit to the dentist. It was something he loved to do.

Ted walked to one corner of the field and I walked to the other picking up blue and gray sweatshirts marking the boundaries. A battered and bruised football, a few players (live bodies will do) and a field with no white lines were ample ingredients for a football game on The Plains. Dusk's shadow slithered across the left side of the field by the maple tree, and covered the grassy middle as Skippy scooped up his white Varsity jacket. The passer-by picked up a stick and dragged it along the side of the road as he headed north toward New Boston Road. Ted and I hopped the ditch and crossed the street looking both ways. He flipped the football from tip to tip with residual nervous energy still pulsing through his body. We walked up the squares of concrete and over the one marked with "D loves P" leading to the front porch. "I wonder what's for supper," Teddy said as he smiled and lightly shoved my shoulder. At that moment, I think I knew what he was thinking—but we didn't talk.

Talk

Talking was pretty much limited to the first layer of skin. We rarely scratched below the surface. Having cancer didn't change Ted's reluctance to tell me what he was thinking. This was no different than before. Especially now though, I tried not to ask too many questions; after all, there were too many of us wanting answers. At first, it was one of us calling him after another. We never knew how many calls he had already gotten in a day. How many calls are too many and how many calls are not enough? Perhaps, my call came at the tail end of one of Jimmy's.

"Hi, Ted, are you going to be home tonight?"

"I'm not sure. Kevin has a game and Brenda and I might go to it."

"I know you two have been running around and back and forth with the chemo and I wondered if you might like me to bring up some supper for you."

"Sure, that sounds good, but you don't have to."

"I know, but I'd like to."

"Well, if you really want to that would be cool. If we're not here we'll leave the house open."

"How's it goin'?"

"No problem. It's goin'."

"Are you havin' any problem eating certain foods?"

"Not really. I can still eat just about anything."

"Okay, I'll see what I can find and maybe I'll make the drive tonight."

"Sure, thanks, but I might not be home."

"I'll take my chances."

There were times when a sense of urgency overcame me, an overwhelming need to be close to Ted, in any way possible. I wanted to see him face-to-face, or hear his voice, or give him a hug. There were times I had the need to do something, anything. I had the need to put thoughts into action. I heard the distant voice of a basketball coach yelling, "Just do something!" It was very frustrating not to know what would or would not be helpful. Sometimes, I had to ask, "Is this helping me or is this helping him?" This was one of those times.

Teddy prided himself on his famous beef stew—that, and the chili he perfected in his crock pot. It was a 70s kind of thing, cooking in a crock pot. Whenever he invited his family up to Loudon to skate on his pond, chili was on the menu.

"The ice is lookin' pretty good and should be set for New Year's. Why don't you plan on coming up?" Teddy gave the hint of a skating party at our family gathering at Christmas.

There was never any formal invitation, either by email or snail mail. There wasn't necessarily a phone invitation either. Most times, the word that Teddy was having everyone up to his house started by someone he had mentioned this to at Christmas. That was Teddy being Teddy. I could never imagine him actually planning a party. It would require too much organizing and way too much fuss.

"Is there anything you would like us to bring?"

"I don't care, I'm makin' chili and we'll have hot dogs and beer. I'm not sure what Brenda's makin'. Don't worry about it. Just come."

We didn't worry about it and we did come, by car loads of cousins with kids, skates, hockey sticks, and winter parkas. The minute I opened the front door, I smelled the pot of hot chili, and had to ask him about his recipe.

"What's your secret Ted?"

"Pigs' tails, puppy dogs' noses, and a pinch of Tabasco. Want to try some?"

"Gee, Ted, you make it sound so enticing. Maybe I'll wait until after I skate."

"Your loss, it might be all gone by then."

"I've lost out with you before."

"What do you mean by that?"

"You know what I mean, don't look so innocent. You always stole my last bite of supper... the one I was saving for last." When we were kids I didn't dare to look up from my plate fearing he would do that trick again. "Cindy, look over there,"—and the perfect piece of roast beef covered with gravy would be gone.

"Is that a fact?" Ted asked as he grabbed his blue ski hat and headed for the back door.

"Yeah it is." I added, following him with my skates in hand.

Even though I wasn't sure I was going to be able to see Ted, my need "to do something" grew stronger throughout the day. After work, I bought some beef stew, an antipasto salad, and some rolls at a local restaurant and left for Loudon. When I got there the house was empty. Too bad, I thought to myself, fearing he wouldn't get home before I would have to leave. I took my time bringing the bags in, one at a time, and then went back to the car to get the cellophane wrapped flowers, which cheered me up even if they didn't anyone else. I stored the salad and beef stew in the refrigerator and started to set the table when a book on the coffee table caught my eye; it was *The Power of Positive Thinking*.

My brother is reading a self-help book—I thought to myself. Things must be more desperate than I thought. I was more familiar with him devouring *The Hobbit*, pages of which were missing, mangled, and marked up from repeated readings. I saw him with his head pushed against the arm of the living room couch holding the book up to his nose, because he was too lazy to go find his glasses. He was so engrossed in his book that he didn't notice the drool sliding from the corner of his lip down to his chin. One of his feet—the one without the sock on it—was on the couch, and the other dangled off the edge, the sock just about ready to fall off. (An uncle nicknamed him "old stockin' foot" because one sock was always slipping off the end of his foot.) He looked so uncomfortable, I thought about getting a pillow to put under his head.

"Ted, you're reading that again?" It puzzled me that he could read the same book over and over. I don't think I've ever read the same book twice.

Slurping up the drool, he answered, "So what, it's a great book. You should try it sometime."

After he finished reading, *The Hobbit* was left behind, squished between two cushions like a left-over pressed sandwich. Lounging on the couch, getting ready to watch TV, I felt a hard lump pressing the cheeks of my butt. It was a pointed corner of *The Hobbit* making its presence known. I reached down between the cushions and pulled it out. With Teddy in mind, I opened to the first page. It had me at, *in a hole in the ground there lived a hobbit*. I couldn't put it down.

On the other hand, I couldn't put *The Power of Positive Thinking* down fast enough. It's not my favorite kind of reading material and I didn't think it was Ted's. It made me so sad to know that Teddy was reading something like it and made me wonder what his reaction was to it, as well as how much of it he had read. Perhaps, I didn't know this side of Ted. Maybe, it was always there, or perhaps, it was new. I left the book where I found it and walked to the kitchen.

Strange, it was, to be walking around my brother's kitchen without him. I invited myself and he said it was fine to come. He told me he would leave the door open and he did. Yet, I didn't visit often, and it felt strange to be at his empty house. I searched through the kitchen cabinets and found dishes, glasses, and silverware and placed them on the dining room table. The gas stove startled me when it suddenly came on, set by a timer. Imagine that, Ted has a gas stove. It made me think, "You've come a long way, baby, to get where you've got to today."

Living in his cramped apartment in Littleton, New Hampshire, he had his standards. Though some may have considered them low standards, Ted considered them his. And, what's wrong with a person setting his own standards? So what if it meant anyone visiting him would have to bring a thermal blanket, wear long underwear and mittens in his living room. He laughed about how many times the water pipes burst. When he came to our house, I watched him shed his layers, first a heavy sweater, then a sweatshirt, then a long sleeve shirt, and finally a t-shirt.

"What's the matter, Ted?" I asked laughing at the pile of clothes mounting on my floor.

Grinning he answered, "It's hot in here."

I found a glass vase in one of the cupboards and began to fix the red and yellow carnations and baby's breath, wondering if Ted and Brenda might surprise me and come home soon. I placed the arrangement in the center of the table, satisfied with the presentation. With nothing left to do, not quite ready to go, I sat at their dining room table and glanced out the glass windows. I thought about his sons Corey and Kevin and all the cousins, and how we played ice hockey on Ted's frozen pond.

Our dad, the "I-played-hockey-for-UNH" father, was showing one of his grandchildren how to skate backwards with a hockey stick in hand.

"Corey boy, grab a stick and let's play some hockey."

On cue, Teddy scooped up a pair of winter boots from the snow-covered shore and tucked them under his arm. Hips swaying left and right, he skated to one end of the pond and threw the boots to the ice. They bounced and slid in opposite directions. Bending over, Ted reached for the boots and spaced them far enough apart to be considered "the net."

Sashaying back to the shore to get another pair, Jimmy slid up behind Ted and slapped his skates with his hockey stick, causing Teddy to trip on a crack in the ice. He lurched forward, wobbled a bit, and then regained his balance.

"Mess with the best and you lay with the rest," Ted yelled over his shoulder as he continued skating.

"Sure, sure, big tough guy," Jimmy taunted back as he went to find the puck.

I laced up my skates and watched as Teddy's skates screeched to a stop, spraying flecks of ice chips on my ski pants.

"You gonna play?" He looked down on me.

"Guess so." I looked up at him.

Field hockey was my sport, ice hockey was not. I was somewhat reluctant, but didn't want to be left out, especially after Ted had asked me to join them. He was relaxed, on his own turf, eager to engage in this winter sport. It was hard to refuse his offer. Like playing football when we were younger, I knew it would feel good.

We chose our sides, family member against family member. Ted and his two boys, Corey and Kevin, joined with my husband Pat (Ted's boyhood buddy) my daughter Mandy, and me. We faced off against Jimmy and his daughter, Jillian, my sister Debbie and her daughters, Emily and Laurie, and my son Matt. Jimmy's youngest son, Jordan, was left to skate on his own.

"Dad, you be the referee," called Debbie.

"I'm not that old," Dad said.

"We know that, but better to be safe than sorry." I backed up Debbie.

Dad was disappointed, but gave in, and we gathered in a cluster in the center of the ice. Dad dropped the round, black puck between Teddy's and Jimmy's slanted hockey sticks. They pounded them up and down on the ice.

"Get it, Ted!" I yelled.

"Get it, Jim!" Debbie yelled.

Jimmy got a solid piece of it and flipped it over to Corey. Corey cradled it and brought it "up ice" with Matt scrambling after him. Catching sight of my son Matt from the corner of his eye, Corey shot the puck over to me. I cradled it for a second before Jimmy snatched it away, hitting me in the shins.

"No roughin' the skater!" I screamed after him.

Dad blew his whistle, "Foul. Two minutes in the penalty box."

Jimmy gave me another poke as he skated over to a tree stump and plunked himself down. He harassed us from the sidelines.

"Mandy's cheatin', she's hangin' aroun' the goal."

Dad ignored Jimmy and kept his eye on Emily. Emily saw the puck flying her way and raised her stick over her shoulder.

"Stickin'!" Dad was getting a good work-out making his calls and keeping up with the game. "Penalty shot. Who's gonna take it?"

Ted was the logical candidate and he skated over near our goal. I cheered him on, "Ted, Ted, he's our man, if he can't do it no one can!" I jumped up, forgetting I was on skates, and landed on my tail bone. Man, that hurt. It did look pretty funny though, and I had to laugh along with the rest of the onlookers, while caressing my aching butt.

Ted scored, then Jimmy, Corey, and Matt—it went back and forth for the whole game—until Dad had to blow his whistle. Jordan, the littlest guy, got clobbered by Laurie who didn't see him fumbling onto the ice with his brand new skates. The game ended in a tie, but not before Teddy got his last say with Jimmy.

Bodies and hockey sticks brushed against each other, but Jimmy thought he had control of the puck. He pushed it out of the hovering pack of skaters and directed it toward his goal. In the confusion, he lost sight of it and was surprised to see Teddy speed skating, leading a round black puck toward his own goal.

"Where the hell did that come from?" Jimmy fired at Teddy. Teddy was already slapping the puck into his goal by the time Jimmy caught up to him. I couldn't figure it out either until I realized what Teddy had done—he had pulled a hidden puck out of his pocket.

"Nice trick, Ted." I smiled at Ted.

"I know. When do you think he'll figure it out?" Ted grinned back at me.

The mysteries confined within the wooden walls, the burgundy draperies, the Oriental rug, and Ted's black, leather recliner did not reveal their secrets. I searched for some clue of understanding of the conversations held in that room. But, I was shut out. Teddy didn't talk about what he was thinking and neither did Brenda. They let me in to the privacy of their home, but not in to their innermost thoughts. I stepped over the curled-up edge of the well-traveled Oriental rug and walked around the coffee table, glancing once more at the self-help and cancer information books left there for examination. My eyes covered the light stained wood of the walls from the rough-hewn beams in the ceiling to the trimmed moldings around the floor, and they had nothing to say to me. My hand touched the soft, black leather of the La-Z-Boy recliner, where Ted spent much of his days watching TV and reading, and it did not speak to me. The gentle waves in the burgundy draperies were as tight-lipped as a brother and sister sworn to secrecy—where secrets would be held safe. It was time for me to go.

I left the same way I came, alone and through the front door, carrying as much baggage with me as I had left behind. Troubled that I had not seen Ted, but satisfied that I had "done something," I tuned in to WOKQ on the ride home. What a switch, Ted and I used to listen to Fleetwood Mac and now I'm listening to Shania Twain. I turned her up as loud as I could stand, *it's bout as bad as it could be...seems everybody's buggin' me up, up, up...*

Complications

A hole in Ted's chest, called a port, was used for inserting the chemotherapy. It eliminated the need for an IV every time he received treatment. After five months into his treatment, it became infected. This was something we were afraid might happen. Mom could hear the disappointment in his voice when he called to tell her about it.

"I'm havin' trouble with the port for my chemo. My arm is sore and swollen."

"What have you done about it?"

"I went to the doctor's last night and he removed the line and the port. He thought there might be a blood clot and an infection."

"What else are they doing for you?"

"They put me on blood thinners and told me to rest."

"And, are you resting?"

Ted may have responded politely but I knew he wanted to scream. Men are not supposed to rest—especially not for months on end. He was tired of being held back and I knew it. That winter, we went for a cross country ski in Maudslay State Park in Newburyport, Massachusetts. Again, I felt the need for us to spend some time together.

Heavy snow storm after heavy snow storm left a good three feet base of snow—ideal for cross country skiing.

"Ted, have you ever been to Maudslay State Park?" I asked excitedly.

"No, never heard of it."

"You've never heard of it? Well, this will be a treat for you. It's known for its wide variety of trees and it overlooks the Merrimack River. It also has a section closed off because of a nesting place for eagles. Want to go cross country skiing there sometime this week? It's one of my favorite places to go." I was eager to show Ted an outdoor place he had never seen before and he agreed to join me.

There were only a few parked cars when we drove into the parking lot. We were the only ones unloading our skis. There were no crowds, no lines, no concession stands, and no fees. I sliced through the silence, pulling my long ski poles from the back end of Pat's black Explorer. Ted started to get out of the car.

"Hey, Ted, not like in the old days when we used to go skiing at the farm and at Wild Cat."

He paused, leaned on the car door, and took in the view. Across the street from the parking lot was an old white building for visitor information, a sign posted with visitor instructions, and fields of rolling hills. A road, lined with parallel ski tracks, led to the Merrimac River. Ten feet tall, overgrown rhododendron bushes hung over the road, burdened with a heavy coat of white snow. Cotton-ball clouds drifted across a light blue sky and two skiers could be seen in the distance, ready to enter the woods. Instead of answering my question, Teddy asked, *who are those miserable persons?*

"I don't know," I laughed. "How dare they invade our space?"

I was still thinking about our rides to Wild Cat, as Ted slowly reached for his skis. Those rides were windy and filled with sharp curves. Depending on the driver, they were enough to make anyone carsick. Ted and I both suffered from motion sickness.

"Remember when you sat in the back of that old station wagon and rode backwards all the way to the mountain?" I asked. (Ted threw up all over the car.)

"Thanks for reminding me…I have plenty of those kinds of moments to remind me all the time now," he said softly.

"Sorry about that, I didn't mean to bring up a sore subject."

"That's all right. Now I know what all my sisters went through when they were pregnant. I guess I never thought much about that."

"Not that we ever wanted you to."

Nausea, I felt, must be the worst thing about having chemo. It sure was the worst thing about being pregnant. Sick people bent over a toilet seat heaving their guts out day after day, never knowing what they'll be able to eat, was an image I couldn't get out of my head. I thought about a Reach-to-Recovery (breast cancer survivor) volunteer that worked for one of our American Cancer Society units. She was optimistic as she shared her experience with me, "Nausea can get pretty bad but it's not as bad as it used to be. They've made a lot of progress with the treatments and people don't get nearly as sick." Thank good medicine for that, but nausea is still nausea.

The sweat that creeps across foreheads and the rumbling in stomachs brought on by chemical reactions can bring the strongest of men to their knees—football players like my brother included—praying to the porcelain God. I attended the funeral of one young man who prayed to the porcelain God, got knocked out by the toilet seat cover, and was asphyxiated on his own vomit in the middle of the night. My grandfather, suffering from the flu, vomited so hard he ruptured his esophagus and died of the infection that followed. I have lain on cold linoleum bathroom floors to make the disrupting, vile sensation go away. Chanting, without speaking, I have repeated over and over, "Make it go away, make it go away, make it go away." As a mother, watching my child hunched over in agony, I wanted the power to make the pain go away. As a sister, I wanted the nausea to go away for Ted.

We tucked our skis under our arms and clomped across the road. Snow stars glistened on the white surface as I threw my skis down and clipped my boots into them. I headed toward the trail before I realized that Ted was just finishing clipping into his first ski. I glanced over my left shoulder, twisted my upper body, and leaned one arm on my ski pole to get a better look. Like a pack horse pulling cement blocks at Deerfield Fair, Ted's every movement was slow and deliberate and carried a ton of weight. Maybe this wasn't such a good idea. Slowly, he raised his body and fumbled with the next binding. Slowly, he bent over to pick up his poles. Slowly, he pushed forward looking in my direction, "So, what's the hold up? Where are we goin'?"

"I thought we would go toward the area that is closed off for the eagles. Maybe we'll get a glimpse of one." I waited until the tip of his ski brushed the end of mine and pointed down the meadow. "How far do you feel like goin'?"

"I don't care. I'll take my time. I'm not as fast as I used to be. Guess I'll have to let you lead the way."

Removing the line and port in Ted's chest meant that his next chemo treatment would have to be done with IV's through his veins, instead of through the medically-made hole in his chest. We thought, at least it was only for one more treatment. Yet, even on blood thinners and antibiotics, his right arm continued to be swollen, and his fingers and hand tingled. Friday, January 17, 2003, he spent the day at the hospital having an obstruction, near the port, removed. By the time he called Mom the next day, he was feeling better, and told her how they took out the obstruction with a "roto rooter."

The snow was good, light-weight but plenty of it. This meant the skiing must be good and we would go to the farm on Sunday afternoons. Dad rounded us up, asking, "Does anyone want to go skiin'?" There may be five or six of us or there may only be two or three, but however many, we scrounged up our ski paraphernalia and started throwing it in the back of the station wagon. Edges of skis hit edges of skis and none of us seemed to care—like colorful pick up sticks—they were left in a disorganized cluster until we were ready to sort them out.

"Hey, I think you've got my poles." I was suspicious of Teddy taking something of mine.

"No I don't. Yours are under that pile. And, where are my black gloves?" He sounded irritated.

There were some items that Teddy cared about. Good ski equipment was one of them. The most excited I ever saw him at Christmas was when he got a brand new pair of stretchy blue ski pants.

"I don't know. I don't have 'em." I was having enough trouble finding my own things.

Finding all personal (I use that term loosely) ski items was a challenge, but even more challenging was putting them together. First, there was the task of getting into ski boots. I sat on the tail end of the station wagon with my mitten-less fingers struggling with the cold. I balanced myself on the lumpy metal while pulling on "pass me down" boots. I teetered back and forth as I tried to tie up the laces. "Shit. My lace just broke again." I glanced toward Teddy who was fastened into his skis and reaching for his poles. "There's always tomorrow for dreams to come true." He called to me as he quickly skied out of sight.

Ted wasn't there to see me fight the mousetrap–like, uncooperative ski bindings. I bent over my ski and stretched the metal spring. I tried to lock my boot into place. Time and time again it snapped back in the opposite direction. My ski bindings gave me enough frustration to make me consider giving up skiing altogether. Teddy talked me out of that. It seemed like forever before I could line my skis in his parallel tracks and follow him down the road to the ski hill.

Ted was scheduled to have his last chemo treatment on Monday, January 20th. On Wednesday, January 22nd, he arrived at the hospital to be told that both his red and white blood cell counts were still too low. He also had chills and a fever. He was given antibiotics by IV and was allowed to go home. The doctors told Brenda they thought the fever was due to the infection in his port. On a positive note, they felt hopeful he may be in remission from the cancer.

Gliding my skis across the snow, I deliberately slowed my pace making sure I didn't get too far ahead of him, aware that I knew that he knew he was not up to speed. We shared the same earthly space, but he was in an entirely different world and one that I could not get into. An activity that should have brought him joy—being outside, being free to ski on freshly fallen snow, and being surrounded by nature's finest trees—was not making him happy. He was having trouble keeping his pants up and tugged at his waist. "I don't have a butt anymore," he complained.

"So what, it was never as cute as mine." I changed the subject, "Man, there sure are a lot of different trees out here. You're the expert. What kind is this one?" I never could identify one tree from another.

"That's a shag bark hickory and over there is a white poplar. White poplars are pretty unusual to see in this part of the country. I like white birches myself."

So near to the end of Ted's first treatment, yet so far away from recovery. On Thursday, January 23rd he was admitted to Concord Hospital—the antibiotics they were using were not working. Nothing was. It was about this time that I remember the tell-tale puckering of Ted's lower lip, and the bracing against his tears that wanted to flow. Months of waiting, months of treatment, and months of hoping did not give Ted the news he so anxiously awaited to hear. It was not necessary to ask him how he was doing. His quivering, voiceless lips did the talking. Upon hospital admission, to make matters worse, he was put in isolation. We were not allowed to visit.

Approaching the ski hill, I could see Teddy's worn, denim jacket covered in snow, and rope burns dug deep into his pockets. Skiing at the farm meant facing the rope toe—something I sweated over. An abandoned, blue and white Chevy was lodged in the snow bank at the bottom of the hill. Our uncle got the engine running so a rope could be attached to a pulley and we could get a ride up the hill. The problem was that this could be fairly tricky. Especially if your older brother or older and more experienced cousins were waiting impatiently in line behind you.

Nervously, I approached the fast-moving rope as Teddy came whizzing in front of me. Trying to get in as many "runs" as possible (the better the skier the more runs in an afternoon) he wasn't about to wait for me to get up my nerve.

"Just grab it and hold on. Let the rope pull you." He yelled back to me as he skied up beside the rope, bent over, grabbed the rope with both hands, and let it yank him forward. He made it look easier than it was.

Like a dog watching a toy train racing around and around on a track, I watched for my moment to attack. I focused in on the thick, tan/brown rope and made my move, grabbing it with both gloves as hard and fast as I could. The rope took on a life of its own, whipping me to the ground. Frantic, with skis criss-crossing under me and poles jabbing me in my sides, I fought to kick myself away from the rope that was burning grooves into my tipped thigh. (Sometimes, the engine had to be stopped so the rope could go limp and allow the downed skier to get untangled.) I managed to get far enough away from the rope in time for Teddy to get ready for his next turn.

"Havin' a little trouble?" He asked, sliding toward me and reaching to help pull me up.

"No. I love gettin' knocked over by that man-eatin' rope."

When Ted's temperature reached one hundred four degrees, a specialist in communicable diseases was consulted. The doctor ordered a chest X-ray and it confirmed that Ted had pneumonia. Ice packs placed under his arms helped to bring his fever down, and he was changed to oral antibiotics. I went to visit him on Sunday, January 26th. I knew it was going to be tough to see him. I tried to think of things I could say, but nothing quite right came to mind. As I rounded the corner of the hall, and passed one of his nurses, I still hadn't thought of anything good to say. Do you say to someone who is at the lowest of low points, "This is just another set back?" How do you know it is just another set back? Jimmy could tell him, "You'll get through this and it will be okay." I couldn't. When I entered his hospital room, he was sitting on the mattress with blankets pulled up to his waist. Ted tried so very hard to force a smile, but he was too near tears to make it look real.

I led Ted to the edge of the eagles' nesting ground and stopped to read the sign, "Do Not Enter." A cloud inched its way across the darkening sky and cast a black shadow over the woods beyond the roped-off path. It was eerily quiet. I imagined Teddy mimicking the cowardly lion—shouting at the top of his lungs, *if I were king of the forest*...and let that memory linger without a mention of it. My eyes traced one side of the path and then the other. The trees were thick with branches spreading in every direction. Wind-swept snow buried the lower bushes. This was a place that had aged with time. People, long passed, had thought to preserve this living, breathing sanctuary. I could feel its heart beating. And, Robert Frost could well have been standing there with us reciting, *two roads diverged in a yellow wood, and sorry I could not travel both.* Or Joyce Kilmer, *I think that I shall never see a poem as lovely as a tree.* I searched the sky for signs of an eagle and then turned to see what Teddy was doing. He was searching, too.

My mom's "mother's intuition" kicked in on Tuesday, January 28th. She was supposed to do her volunteer work as a retired nurse at Bakie Elementary School, but thoughts of Ted consumed her. She needed to get to the hospital. When the school nurse called to say she didn't have to come in she was relieved. Mom called and cancelled her morning coffee with church friends and made plans to go to Concord. Her sister offered to join her.

Together they drove to Concord Hospital and arrived about 11:00 after the doctors had made their morning rounds. A CT scan the day before confirmed what Ted had dreaded to hear; the cancer was back. The cancer "was back." I had to wonder, had it ever actually gone away? The fevers brought the cancer raging forward. Teddy knew his body, and he knew what the fevers were telling him. He knew they weren't from an infection. He didn't need an "M.D." after his name to figure that out. He just hoped that they were smarter than him. Mom took Ted in her arms and they cried together like they had never cried together before.

My frozen thighs, stinging from my wet dungarees, made me acutely aware it was time to head back to the farmhouse. The sandpaper-like material was beginning to chafe my skin. Dark blue streaks tracing a pattern up the snow-covered hill made me realize my new dungarees hadn't yet faded to a proper light-blue denim hue. White strands of cotton formed the shape of an eye and Teddy's bright red knee blinked at me through the hole in his Levi's. He was oblivious. He wanted to keep skiing.

"I'm ready to quit. Are you comin'?"

"Not yet."

"I wanna' get ready to watch *The Wizard of Oz* at Gram's."

This was a big event. Gram and Grampa Bodwell had a new color TV; the first in our family. We were going to get to watch *The Wizard of Oz* in color for the first time. It was only shown once a year and Teddy and I would wait, checking the calendar in anticipation. This year would be extra special.

"I'll be there," Teddy assured me as he grabbed hold of the rope and counted his last run. I slid the rest of the way down the hill and

Kathy skied over to join me. We had had our fill. Distant cows bellowed from the bowels of the barn and beckoned us in from the cold. Like highlighted lines in a treasured book, tangerine streaks stretched across the horizon, marking the change in the day.

Ted was told that he needed to have a PET scan, which is more conclusive than a CT scan, which is more conclusive than an X-ray, which is more conclusive than blood work. From one test, to another test, to another, the thought of Ted being a guinea pig had the ring of truth—yes, it rang true. I began to wonder, how many tests must Ted have before he is allowed to be free? The answer, my friend, was circulating in his cells. He had the PET scan on Friday, January 31st.

A pile of boots, mittens, and hats mounted in the hallway as each of us dropped our wet clothing and entered Gram's kitchen. The smell of home-baked desserts lingered in the air and sucked us in. I surrendered to the glass dish placed on the checkered tablecloth piled high with brown squares of Gram's famous fudge. The luxury of biting into rich chocolate melting in my mouth was enough to make me forget about the tingling sensation in my near-frost-bitten fingers. I liked to press a small ball of the fudge between my tongue and the roof of my mouth and let it seep into my pores. My numb fingers itched with a new sensation as I licked away the sugar.

Wednesday, February 5th, Ted got the results of the PET scan. As suspected, they were not good. The "old tumors" were gone but two new tumors were seen in his lower back. There was talk of going to Dartmouth-Hitchcock Medical Center.

"I got the couch," Kathy claimed running into the living room.

"Me too." I was on her heels and so were a few others.

We guarded our territory knowing that Teddy might try to push us out when he came in. We wanted to be comfortable when the movie started, but Teddy had his ways. He flipped his wet woolen sock off the end of his foot and hung it in front of our faces. Raising his right eyebrow he growled like a German commander, "You vil move or I vil haff to slap you silly with this vet sock. Don't make me hurt you." Squished against the couch cushions, three of us squealed and covered our faces. It would take more than his command to make us give up the couch. He carried out his threat and began slapping us with his sock—dirty from being dragged across the farm-beaten floor. A lump of crystallized snow, clinging precariously from soaked yarn, scraped across my eyelid. I jumped off the couch and grabbed a loose pillow.

The doctors in Concord consulted with the Norris Cotton Cancer Center (NCCC) at Dartmouth-Hitchcock Medical Center in Hanover, New Hampshire. I was familiar with the NCCC. A few years earlier, I had visited it as a representative from the American Cancer Society (ACS). In my professional navy blue suit and red knit sweater, I proudly sat in on the presentation of one of the researchers who was partially funded by the ACS. At the time, I remember being very impressed, even though I couldn't fully appreciate much of what he said. It sounded fascinating.

As Teddy continued to wield his wet, dirty sock, I pounded him on the back with a red, puffy pillow. He flicked his thumb and index finger together on the tip of his shoulder, and looked back at me faking his pain, "Ooo, ooo. What's this I feel, a pesky, little mosquito?" I whacked him as hard as I could with my pillow but it only made him laugh. As I lifted my light-weight pillow for another blow, he quickly punched it out of my hands, and sent it flying across the room. It bounced off a gold-trimmed mirror. Teddy had me in a full nelson when we heard Grampa's stern voice calling from the kitchen.

"Hey, settle down in there." A hush passed from one grandchild to the next until we all fell into line. We knew better than to have him say that more than once. Gram and Grampa's souvenir cook-coo clock began to chime. The rooster chirped from out of its hiding place. It was a friendly note that it was 7:00 PM, time for *The Wizard of Oz*.

Their Website sounded reassuring: "The Center treats patients with all forms of cancer, in bright and welcoming facilities that create a positive environment for cure and recovery." I knew there were excellent doctors at the NCCC. Well-educated staff was specialized in cancer therapy. There was cutting-edge research going on there. I also knew there were no guarantees. Not everyone made it out of there alive.

Belly down, I lay on the multi-colored braided rug. With elbows pointed out, I crossed my hands over my pillow and dug my chin into the V of my fingers; a position that would only be comfortable for a short time. Kathy snuggled into an overstuffed chair in the corner and pulled Gram's handmade afghan framed with black yarn over her legs. Her big toe poked through a hole in one of the squares and tickled the arm of another cousin in the next chair. As Dorothy and Auntie Em gathered by the pig's pen, Teddy retrieved his dirty sock and began to roll it into a ball. He took aim and fired it across the living room. It bopped me off the back of my head.

Into the Woods

When the oncologists at Dartmouth Hitchcock asked Brenda how many people to expect at Ted's conference, she answered, "a lot." It was scheduled for February 24, 2003. Brenda knew all of Ted's six siblings and spouses would want to be there. Our parents and Ted's two sons would also need to be there. If all were able to make it there would be a total of eighteen, including Ted and Brenda. Pat and I got there first and waited for the others. As more and more of us arrived, we began to shuffle around the lobby of the Norris Cotton Cancer Center. Staff members came by and greeted us and then scurried away. Apparently, there was confusion about which room we were supposed to meet in. They scrambled to find a larger conference room.

Dr. Cravits, the head of the Oncology Department, was the senior member of Ted's oncologist team. He had a round face and warm eyes—he was average height for a man. Dr. Cravits sized-up this group of family members, tucked in elbow to elbow, and started the meeting by saying, "I guess Brenda wasn't kidding when she said there would be a lot of family." We chuckled in response. Then he got down to business. He gave a summary of Ted's course of treatment thus far and began to review the prospective plan. "What we are proposing is an autologous stem cell transplant."

My eyes traveled the long distance of the black conference room table, scanned four sisters, a younger brother, and reached the cancer-worn face of our older, older brother. Like Boo Radley, who would rather be left behind the door, Ted was forced into the limelight. Everyone's eyes were directed toward him. He was the focus, the attention, and the concern. The details of this meeting were all about him. In reality, I was surprised that he had even given his permission for all of us to be there. This wasn't in his nature. This was not real. But then, I had to ask, "What was his nature?"

Ted was seventeen when he packed a large duffle bag and headed off on an Outward Bound excursion. I wrote in my diary— "Track Practice... I started making my dress... Teddy left for Outward

Bound"—on April 1, 1971. That was it. Those three lines described events in my life. At fifteen, all I knew was that Outward Bound was some kind of special program for selected kids to get some kind of "outdoor education." Our church minister was familiar with this program and spoke to his Pilgrim Youth Fellowship group about it. He asked who would be interested in going. Ted responded. I'm sure with very few words. Reverend Howard endorsed Teddy and gave him the support he needed to get into the program.

My husband had done his research (not a surprise to anyone in the family) before arriving at the Dartmouth Hitchcock meeting. Pat typed up a list of headings and under each heading he jotted down some questions:

Previous Treatment

Stage four at onset of diagnosis?

What caused the initial diagnosis to be incorrect for so many months? Flu symptoms.

Was initial treatment intense enough? Was correct stage determined?

Norris Cotton

Chemo types: how many are you licensed for, how do you determine correct chemo mixture?

Do you tissue test individuals, empirical data?

Are metrics to success rate available?

How many "clean rooms?"

Treatment

Which treatment is preferred for Ted? Why?

Allogeneic: Should donors be screened now? Harvest now?

Are you planning to harvest both blood and marrow?

Recovery Period

Autologous period (6 months?)

Allogeneic period (2 years?)

What are the differences? Different preference for Hodgkins and non Hodgkins, why?

Nutrition and vitamins

What is the ability to absorb nutrition, during treatment period, afterwards?

This is only a sample of the questions Pat put together; there were many, many more.

Looking over his well-prepared list, I felt remiss; I hadn't come with a single question.

I learned that Outward Bound is a program based on the belief that education must come from experiential learning. Teddy was presented a set of challenges that were meant to test his intellect as well as his character. In 1971 as well as today, Outward Bound seeks to discover young adults' innate abilities and to have the students of this program acknowledge responsibility to others in their communities. Learning through outdoor activities and hands-on tasks was something Teddy could relate to. Ted was up for the challenge.

Dr. Bates was young, tall and athletic looking. He stood by Dr. Cravits at one end of the conference room. The two of them didn't try to hide their concern. They were upfront, honest, and informative. Yet, at times, I half-expected one of them to use a familiar Vermont expression, "Hard sayin', not knowin'." They could give the facts based on previous experience, but they could not give reassurance for the myriad of unknowns Ted faced. It was educated guess work on their part.

As Dr. Cravits recounted the history of Ted's case, he noted that Ted was always in the "worst case scenario" of each facet. "He was stage four when he was diagnosed. He is older than the typical age we see with this type of Hodgkin's lymphoma. We would have expected to see more improvement at this point. The chemo he's had should have worked by now." Dr. Cravits paused for a moment, dropped his head, and then lifted it up slowly, "Ted will need a miracle." Though spoken ever so softly, none of us asked him to repeat his words.

After the long litany of negatives going against Ted, he did go on to point out the positives. "On the bright side...we have seen miracles. Ted has taken good care of his body, and was healthy at the onset of his disease. He never smoked and has always exercised. He has a strong heart and this bodes well for him." Dr. Cravits managed a smile as "bodes well for him" left his mouth. Dr. Bates, with all the professional muster he could gather, followed up with, "Ted's a remarkable guy." On that note, there was a collective sigh of agreement.

Teddy was never afraid of a physical challenge, but Outward Bound presented more than that. How much more—I was never really sure. I do know that it made an impression on both of us. He was gone for a month, as I noted in my diary on May 2, 1971: "Saw Teddy for the first time in 4 weeks." He was excited, not boastful, as he described his outdoor adventure.

"They made us sleep overnight by ourselves, with a little bit of food and no one around to help us. We had a compass and had to figure out how to get back to our group leader in the morning. One girl chickened out."

"Why?"

"Well," he paused to reflect, "It was pretty tough. Bein' sent out in the middle of nowhere, in the middle of the woods, and bein' expected to sleep through the night was a lot. It was quite a test for everyone. She couldn't handle it and sent up a flare for one of the counselors."

"That's too bad."

"I know. To top it off she was her own worst enemy. She wasn't much for getting along with people to begin with, and this only made it worse. I felt bad for her."

"I can see why."

"And the snow was wicked deep. It was pretty hard to carry our backpacks through that stuff. About halfway through the trip, she stumbled so many times, me and a few other guys had to help carry her load."

"I bet that didn't go over very well."

"It didn't. And as if that wasn't bad enough, she was kind of goofy-acting and an easy mark to get picked on. I tried to help her out as much as I could, but there wasn't much I could do."

"It's amazing she made it through at all."

"It sure is."

I found it odd that Teddy told me more about the trouble this girl had, than what happened to him. The fact that he told me this much is evidence that the experience affected him. When Teddy told the story about the girl, he was telling a lot about himself. Perhaps some of his compassion for her came from his own experience with being vulnerable. He was all too familiar with being teased for drooling, mixing up his words, and having one sock dangling off the end of his foot. Teddy wasn't nicknamed "old stockin' foot" for nothing.

"Do any of you have any questions?" Dr. Cravits took a break from his talking and looked around the room. I think we were all just trying to absorb as much information as we could. Dr. Cravits continued as we concentrated on the terminology—stem cells, autologous, allogeneic, and platelets.

"If we do an autologous stem cell transplant it means we will take Ted's stem cells from his blood or bone marrow, treat it to kill the cancer cells, and then give those treated cells back to him. We hope those treated stem cells will reproduce new healthy cells and Ted will eventually become cancer free. If we did an allogeneic transplant, we would use a donor's bone marrow or peripheral blood to accomplish the same thing. One reason we try to stay away from allogeneic transplants is because of potential side effects. We're proposing to go with an autologous transplant for Ted."

I tried to stay focused on what the doctor was saying, but it all sounded so much like a guessing game. My mind drifted to a distant Christmas.

"You go hide," Teddy snickered as he nudged me out of the living room.

I did as I was told and left without putting up a fuss. I had to wait in the "middle room" until he would allow me to come back. It would only take a few minutes. While I fiddled with some green and red wrapping paper, Teddy searched our Christmas tree tucked in the corner to the left of the fireplace. He reached around the back of the tree on the side facing our neighbor—a distantly related aunt that lived on the other side of us. Teddy unscrewed one of the light bulbs and the tree went black.

"You can come back now," he hollered from the darkened living room.

I rushed across the braided rug and up to the Christmas tree. I felt the sting of green needles brushing against my belly, as I reached for a bulb at the tip of my fingers. Slowly, I tested a red bulb, then a green one, and then a yellow one. None of them made the lights turn back on.

"You're getting hot," Teddy gave me a hint as I got closer to the unscrewed bulb around the back.

I felt for a loosened bulb and knew it was the chosen one. I tightened the green glass in the socket and stood back in awe as the string of lights brightened the corner. The multi-colored lights and the lit fireplace cast shadows on the pale, yellow stenciled wall. I smelled the natural scent of evergreen. Presents spilled out from under the branches. *Bright colored packages tied up with string.* These were a few of my favorite things. It was a New Hampshire, Norman Rockwell moment.

I turned to Teddy with satisfaction and said, "Your turn to go hide."

We'd had an hour and a half crash course in cancer clinical trials. The information needed to be digested. There was more at stake here than cramming for an exam. Some of us had a better capacity to understand the complex details than others. I wanted to ask an intelligent question, but was afraid it wouldn't come out right. Clasping my hands under the table, I remained silent. I knew as soon as I got out of the room, someone would ask me a question that I wouldn't have the answer to. Secretly, I thanked God when my husband raised his hand.

"How do you treat marrow and blood cells to reduce the percentage of cancer cells?" Pat asked.

"Radiation is the preferred method," replied Dr. Cravitz.

"What is your basis for choosing to go with autologous over allogeneic?" Pat wanted to know.

"We feel, given Ted's current condition and his history, that an autologous transplant would give him the best outcome. We've consulted with other cancer centers and we feel this is the route to go. An allogeneic transplant has the higher risk associated with graft versus host complications. We don't want to risk that if we don't have to."

Life is filled with risk. We all know that. It's a matter of degrees. While I was busy playing kickball, baseball, and attending track practice, Teddy was tromping through the back woods of New Hampshire in freezing temperatures. His Outward Bound excursion was filled with group challenges, individual challenges, and a bit of survival techniques thrown in for good measure. Who knows what kind of inspiration he picked up while he was out there? Ted did not measure the meaning—he did not delay. He did not waste the day.

"What was it like to sleep in the woods by yourself?" I asked, intrigued.

"It was really pretty cool. I had my down sleeping bag, which kept me warm enough and the stars were out that night. It got pretty cold though. I heard a few animals in the distance but nothing too scary. Actually, it was kind of peaceful. I would do it again if I had the chance."

He didn't bring home any photos. I developed my own pictures in my mind. In them, I saw Ted taking on the wilderness, making peace with knee-high snow, plotting his destiny with a compass crammed in between his food rations. The images were ones that made me want to put on a pair of snow shoes and make the same tracks.

"Should Ted's siblings be tested for possible donors?" asked Pat.

"We are considering that, but we are not at that point quite yet," said Dr. Cravitz.

There is no doubt in my mind that each of us wanted to be the perfect match. If asked, we would gladly run to the lab and have our blood tested. When Pat's words filtered through the air and connected with my thought waves, I understood their meaning. It was conceivable that the next step in this crazy world of treatments for Ted's cancer was that his siblings would be checked to see whose blood would be compatible. If the doctors went that far, we all wanted to be prepared. His was a good question. Unfortunately, the doctors deflected the question for the time being. Pat wanted more answers.

"Will visitors be allowed after the transplant?" Pat asked.

"Yes. There will be precautions, such as wearing masks, gloves, and washing of hands before entering his room. If anyone has a cold or flu symptoms, they will be asked to stay away. Also, we don't allow plants, flowers or fresh fruit to be brought in to his room," added Dr. Cravitz.

"What about books?" asked Jimmy.

"Yes. He can have books but they should be new or at least sanitized," replied Dr. Bates.

"How long will Ted have to be in isolation?" asked my brother-in-law, Dave.

"About five to six weeks. We'll provide a stationary bike in his room for him to use as he is able. We recommend daily physical activity whenever possible," said Dr. Bates softly, slowly, and deliberately. I could see by his expression, Dr. Bates was deeply concerned for Ted. It was obvious to me, and perhaps my siblings would agree, that being involved with Ted's case was affecting Dr. Bates.

Ted and I went on a co-ed camping trip sponsored by our church. (It was the summer after Ted's Outward Bound experience.) It seemed strange to be going off to camp with my brother. We had both been away on different camping trips in junior high, but never together. This was a first. Although we were separated into different groups, I was very much aware of his presence. I looked for him during meal times. I think the reason he agreed to go was because the camp program promised to have a good amount of outdoor activities, like camping in the woods, ropes courses, hiking, and boating, all things in which he excelled.

Instead of sitting around the campfire contemplating the creation of the universe, Teddy made the campers, and himself, laugh. He flexed his chest muscles up and down in rhythmic fashion. It was fun to watch Teddy abandon his usual self-consciousness. His picture-perfect, straight white teeth were flashed on those who were fortunate enough to be in on one of his jokes. We were around kids who didn't know us, didn't have preconceived expectations, and didn't judge us by past behaviors. (It was much the same as it was for Brenda and me during a different church camp experience.) Running through these woods—unfamiliar as they were—Teddy was able to appreciate every bit of stress put on his body. He took any mental tests in stride. He reveled in the fatigue that settled in at the end of each day. His muscles were pushed to the limit.

The three-sided, brown log dining cabin faced the lake. Campers gathered there for breakfast and supper. Lunch was usually spent somewhere out in the woods, along a stream, or at a look-out point in one of the trails. Approaching the dining cabin meant navigating tree limbs that hadn't been cut and dragged away from the path and giant roots. Any number of jagged rocks and lumps of dirt lay in wait for an unconscious camper. I was one of them. On my way to breakfast one morning I sang, unaware of what awaited me on the path, "So high can't go over it, so low can't go under it, so big can't go round it, must go through the door…" One of those obstructive roots reached up from the ground, grabbed me by my ankles, and sent me sprawling face first into a pile of rotting leaves. Spitting leaves out of my mouth and dusting myself off, I glanced up to see Teddy wiping milk from his chin. He just rolled his eyes and shook his head. Hobbling toward him, I could feel my lower lip beginning to swell.

"That lip's gonna look pretty good by the time we get home. At least you can't blame it on me."

"Wanna make a bet? I can tell everyone that you lost in arm wrestling and took it out on me."

"They'd never believe you."

He was probably right. Instead of trying to make a point, I asked, "Are you doin' the solo overnight?"

Every camper was given the option of taking a sleeping bag, a book of matches, some food, some mosquito repellent, a flashlight, and finding a place in the woods to sleep overnight by themselves. It was risky to go out alone and it was buggy, but it wasn't real risky. Yet, this was my chance to see what it was like to sleep alone in the woods, in June under the stars. I was looking forward to it.

"Me and my buddies have already checked out some cool places. I want to sleep near one of the cliffs overlooking the lake."

"I've been out lookin' too, but I haven't found a good place yet."

"Just make sure it's dry." Teddy glanced back over his shoulder as he left for his camp site. "Good luck…see ya, wouldn't wanna be ya."

I spent the next hour scouting through the woods to find a good place to sleep. I was too chicken to go too far away from my routine camp site, which limited my options. The place I finally decided on was nothing special. The spot was surrounded with trees and the ground covered with moss, decaying leaves, and rocks with bits of mica.

My mom was brave enough to ask what had been on her mind, "Ted has always had a high bilirubin count. Could this have anything to do with his cancer?"

"That's an interesting question, Mrs. Clark. I'm not sure if we have any way of telling whether that could be a factor or not. I'm not aware of any connection," Dr. Cravitz said.

"What about the recovery period?" Jimmy wanted to know.

"Because the immune system is so compromised, there's always concern for infection. People should continue to stay away if they have any cold or flu symptoms. His diet will need to be monitored as he will be pretty weak for awhile. He'll know best what he will be able to do. There will be continued tests and we'll set up visits with a visiting nurse."

"What about testing his sons for a possible match?" Jimmy asked.

"We're considering that also," Dr. Cravits paused, "but normally we don't like to use a child's blood. It is not recommended." He did not need to go into detail. The implied, "if Ted were to die," could leave a devastating effect on any donor. It was especially troubling to think about how Kevin or Corey might feel.

Behind family doors, Ted toyed with his son, Kevin. With his morbid sense of humor, he'd sneak up behind him, tickle his boy's neck, and taunt, "Kev, Kev, you'll be the chosen one." Knowing that Kevin was afraid of needles, Ted couldn't resist the temptation of teasing his son; in the same way he rubbed his dog's fur in a backward direction or gave me a "noogie." That's when he took one of his knuckles and scraped it across the top of my head. He was prone to minor acts of torture. It was another example of Teddy being Teddy. It was his way of "playing."

Corey and Kevin sat across the table from me. Corey was fighting the flood of emotions the doctors' words about his dad brought into his young life. This pressure had been building up for months and threatened to burst at any minute. It was pressure coming from within that forced him to be a man and to be there for his dad. External pressures were also in the room—the doctors, his grandparents, and all his aunts and uncles wondering how he was handling the situation. He didn't move a muscle. His youthful eyes, filled with angst, were attentive. I knew his father was glad to have him there.

Kevin, the younger of the two, was more visibly stricken. His flushed red cheeks showed in bright contrast to his pale, white complexion. His handsome, deep brown eyes were marred with traces of red. He looked more like a man-child than a boy. The months of having a sick father around the house, doctor visits, and disappointing news had taken its toil. Kevin's childhood was eclipsed with his dad's cancer. He, too, became the focus of our thoughts. I wondered what this was doing to him. Like his brother, he did not move a muscle.

I retraced my earlier steps, as I prepared for my night in the woods. I saw a piece of mica embedded in a piece of granite. It reminded me of climbing Mount Chocorua with Dad, Teddy, and Jimmy. Midway up the trail, Dad threw Jimmy on his shoulders and coaxed us along.

"How much farther is it?" I asked.

"It's not that far," Dad answered, "Why don't you and Teddy see who can find the biggest piece of mica."

"What's mica?" I asked.

"It looks like shards of broken mirror plastered to rocks." He searched the path until he found a good chunk and scraped it off the side of a large rock with his pocket knife. He held it up for us to see. Dad's black and blue thumb (hit many times over by a hammer) moved gently as he peeled away the layers of mica. He pulled them apart like sheets of tissue paper.

"Crystals are split into thin sheets that are tough yet flexible. These sheets are reflective, reactive, and chemically inert." Dad reverted back to his chemistry class.

"Let's stop with the chemically-inert stuff and get goin'," Teddy said as he elbowed Dad in the side.

"All right, all right. But, someday you might thank me for that information."

"Yeah. When I'm on my next million dollar mica expedition?"

"Ha ha. I bet you can't find any." Dad put his hands on his hips and arched his back, "Whoever finds the biggest piece of mica will get a prize at the top of the mountain."

"There's a giant piece right over there!" Teddy pointed off in the distance and ran toward a huge boulder with a crack running up the middle. A shiny reflection had caught his eyes. When he got there he realized it was a piece of plastic wrap that had adhered to the wet surface. With his back to us, he scooped up the piece of wrap and tucked it in his pocket.

"Let me see. Let me see." I hurried over.

"Not gonna show yeah till we get to the top." He was convincingly smug.

All the way to the top we scoured the mountain side for pieces of mica. Dad put Jimmy down and he tried to keep up. I found a very small piece, about the size of a quarter that was not very impressive. I gave up on my chance of a prize. Teddy never did find any real mica, but he was first to get to the top.

Wind blew strands of my loose brown hair across my nose and lips—I brushed them away. A daring hiker, lying on his belly close to the edge of the peak, banged two rocks together. It made an echo travel into the valley. We all made it to the summit and it was time to see who had the largest piece of mica.

"Come on, Teddy, let's see yours." I tugged at his hooded gray sweatshirt.

"Not until you guess how big it is."

"Is it bigger than that rock?" I pointed at a small rock.

"Oh yeah."

"Is it as big as a card?" I rumpled the bottom of my shorts.

"Nope."

"Is it the size of my fist?" I made a small fist.

"You'll never guess so I'll just have to show you."

With a chuckle, he pulled the fake piece of mica out of his pocket.

Like the end of a grueling poker game, all the cards were on the table; any question that any family member had been able to ask was out there. We had had our chance to speak. The doctors were patient, and thorough, and as honest as they could be. As Mom would later say, "They did not minimize the serious problems ahead." I couldn't help thinking about other meetings that Ted's doctors needed to attend. There were others that needed their help. It was commendable that they spent this quality time with us and we appreciated their efforts. At least there was a plan. We all knew if this plan didn't work, there may or may not be another meeting like this one.

I remember thinking how incredible it was that Teddy sat through this intensive meeting which was all about him and remained composed. He was involved but restrained. He was hurting but feeling. He was thinking but not saying too much. At times, he smiled up at one or another of us. He looked to be on the verge of tears. His emotion was readable. The number of people there, the questions asked, and the nature of the truth about what was happening was something I could never imagine him allowing to take place. Yet, I think he was "getting used to" this kind of prying into his personal life. He was beginning to say and do things that I didn't think were possible. Ted's way of being in the world was changing but he was still a man of action. This meeting was reassuring because it confirmed that there was a plan. There was something more that Ted could do. He began to mentally prepare himself for the stem cell transplant.

When I set out in the woods with my sleeping bag, book of matches, flashlight, candy bar, and mosquito repellant—Teddy was with me—he moved through me. In my mind, I always thought, "If Teddy can do it then I can too," even if it didn't always prove to be true. I resolved to go down trying.

Alone, I faced the darkness. The warmth of the sun had left for the day. I pulled a heavy, dark green sweatshirt down over my blue and white striped turtle neck. Like faux fog seeping across a stage, shadows replaced light spots as I continued to retrace my steps. I inspected the ground for tripping sticks as I passed the moss-covered tree stump. Mom would love that patch. I continued to the left of the clump of birches, then up a bit of incline, and searched for the massive oak with a branch that had been split by lightening. It looked like it was about to break off—but it was still hanging in mid-air. The blackness of night was filling in the spaces between the tall trees.

My family filed out of the conference room like the show of cards had proved to be unmistakably bad. We bowed our heads and shuffled our feet. Together, but silently, we struggled to regain our composure. We planned to drive to my older sister Muffy's and her husband Dave's house to drown our sorrows in pizza and beer. I reached the door at the same time as Brenda.

I envied Brenda on "Mommy Larson's" kindergarten playground for her long, thick, beautiful black hair pulled back in a ponytail. I envied her for Paul Robb liking her instead of me—for her getting the part of Peter Cottontail's mother when I got stuck as a head of cabbage in the vegetable garden. She surpassed me with every math test and was bold enough to ask me what I got. If all that wasn't enough, she took the leading role in the fourth grade play. As Johnny Appleseed's mother—she did her best acting. I pouted, amazed with the rest of the audience at her performance. When she came down with strep throat the week before, I eagerly began to practice as her stand-in but she recovered in time to go on with the show.

Coming out of the conference, I couldn't stand in for her now either. She was staring as Ted's wife, a role that was having its difficulties. She was the only one who could play this part. Though I had my own thoughts, Brenda would need to call the shots. I would need to support decisions that she and Ted made. One of their decisions was should Ted have an autologous stem cell transplant or an allogeneic stem cell transplant? I'm sure there were days that she would have liked someone else to fill in for her, but she had to go on with life. Brenda had two high school-aged boys, a full-time job with the State of New Hampshire, as well as her husband and herself to worry about. This wasn't easy. Running was her salvation.

For as long as I have known Brenda, there are still mysteries that separate us and secrets that we have not shared. There was a time when we stayed up late in her camper-trailer, parked in the backyard. She talked about pressing things on her mind. But now, we seemed so far apart. Things change. Why had we not seen more of each other over the years? Why did I know so little of what she was feeling? Why didn't she want to confide in me? It's not that we ever argued. Perhaps, it is that we had gone our separate ways. Perhaps, we had separated a long time ago and I had tried to hold onto the past. My perception, skewed as it may have been, was that our shared childhood and adolescence were defining connections. I thought what we shared in the past would set our relationship apart from those in the rest of my family, but maybe I was wrong.

Our past was filled with memories. There were pajama parties with her doing most of the talking and me falling asleep, and walks along Salisbury Beach in the early morning hours while the trash collectors tried to pick *us* up. They thought I was a freshman in college and she was my little sister. There were hikes in the White Mountains and staying overnight at Craig Camp—at ages fifteen, twenty, twenty-five, and thirty. As my brother did for me, I led the way. We played basketball together. I scored while she set the picks for me. I think I'm beginning to see the answer.

Perhaps, Brenda was tired of trying to compete with me. She, like Ted, needed her space, her own place, her own identity. Like going away to church camp where no one there knows you; you can be yourself, or be who you feel you want to be, or find a comfort zone that is right for you. We all need a comfort zone.

Some boys "marry their mother." Some girls "marry their father." My friend Brenda "married my brother." Brenda traded a childhood of competition with me to adulthood of competition with her husband. Some of these competitions she won. Some he won. Competition can be a good thing, but when is too much competition enough? Friends of the "Ted and Brenda" couple saw Teddy whizzing along in bike races, always at the front of the pack, while his wife huffed and puffed behind him, determined to succeed. In the long run, she did. She took her running seriously and began to train for triathlons. In the past, we ran road races together, me in front and her trailing behind. Today, I couldn't even come close to her on my best day! Things change.

So, when we met at the conference-room doorway, there was a lot of history behind us. As if we were two awkward five-year-olds meeting at the sand-filled sailboat at Mommy Larson's for the first time, we were unsure about what to do. To hug each other was not a familiar act. In our "WASP" nature, we were more used to keeping a culturally accepted distance. Today, however, hugging seemed to be in order. Not obligatory, this hug was a knee-jerk reaction. Filled with uncertainty but going with my gut, I wrapped my arms around her petite frame. She responded in kind. Her multi-shades of brown/black hair mixed with streaks of gray, mingled with my freshly dyed, brown hair. Tears formed as we continued to embrace. I hoped my thoughts could be conveyed through osmosis. I asked, "Are you going back to Muffy's?"

I unrolled my dark green sleeping bag lined with soft, red, plaid cotton and patches of sticky pine pitch. Kids thought it was funny to fill each other's sleeping bag with pine needles when no one was looking. I ran my fingers over the rough ground to make sure it was dry and felt for sharp rocks that would stick into my back in the middle of the night. A white pillow case was filled with my "safety kit" and I tucked it inside my bag. I took off my orange-colored shit kickers (same style, but different size than Ted's) and placed them outside my bag. As if getting ready for a "sack race," I wrestled my way into my sleeping bag, still wearing all my daytime clothes. I flicked my flashlight on and off, and made a sweep of my surroundings before placing it under cover by my right shoulder. I rested on my back, my head on my flimsy white pillow, and felt a twig inching its way toward my neck. I fluffed the pillow up and repositioned it several times before getting everything just right.

Inhaling and exhaling the cool summer air, I could hear myself breathing. I tilted my head back and clasped my hands under my neck. I gazed upward. This was a banquet fit for a nature lover, and I feasted on the black night sky scattered with shiny, bright stars. My eyes guided my memory back to a time when Teddy and I were much, much younger.

"Come on, Cindy; help me take out the trash." I wondered why a healthy, strong, twelve-year-old boy needed his little sister to trudge through the snow, in the cold and dark of this winter night, to burn the trash. Besides, it was his job, not mine. I had my own chores to do. And, he never helped me with mine; at least not that I could think of.

"No, I don't want to." I tried to be firm.

"Come on, we'll name the stars." He used his most persuasive tone and I knew I was doomed. I went to put on my rubber boots.

Side-by-side we walked through the snow. I glanced at the ground and noticed that he didn't have his boots on.

"Where are your boots?" I asked.

"I don't know. It's not gonna take very long. Why bother?"

I thought about how cold his feet must be as the tip of my nose began to turn red. We dragged the collected bags of trash, way in back of our house, by the edge of the snow-covered garden. We dumped the paper scraps and cardboard cereal boxes into the rusted barrel. Teddy struck a match and then threw it into the debris sticking over the rim. We watched the tips of red, yellow, and orange flames consume the colorful Fruit Loops box and lick the air above it. We warmed our hands and stood a safe distance. Teddy and I posed with our heads tilted back pondering the sky. The magic of the vast, star-filled sky was so powerful in its chemistry that even two young children paused to appreciate its presence. We picked out our favorite brightest stars.

"Up there, that one is Aunt Harriet," Ted said. Naturally, he went first.

"Is that the same one you named the last time?" I asked skeptically.

"I don't remember, just name another one."

"Okay, that one over there is Great Grandpa Simeon."

I woke up from my sleep in the woods—refreshed and well-rested. When I saw Teddy at breakfast, he shot me a glance.

"How did it go last night?"

"Great, just great." I cut it short. He wouldn't want to hear a long story about it.

"Hey, do you remember that game we used to play when we took out the trash? We used to name the stars after people who died."

Nothing Can Stop It

It crawls. It creeps. It eats you alive. Ted's cancer was like *The Blob*. Steve McQueen used a flame thrower on *The Blob* to make it stop its destruction. I thought of the game Pac Man to describe Ted's cancer's vicious consumption of human life form—Ted thought of *The Blob*.

Teddy wrote a computer note to himself, "*How do you kill a Tumor, You are going to have to do it yourself. Like in the matrix when Leo finds out he is the one, and jumps into the body of a sentinel and blows it up...Every time I give myself a shot of Lovinnox, I'm really injecting a tumor buster into the bastard...The tumor is like the movie the blob, where Steve McQueen, takes care of it with a flame thrower.*"

This is what I was looking for when he was alive. This is what I discovered after he was gone. This is what Ted thought of his cancer. I'm surprised he didn't mention James Bond, hero of the Ian Fleming books that were strewn all over his teenage bedroom. Surely 007, his favorite action character of all times, could have devised a tumor-killing devise. Or, maybe he could have called on the services of Dr. No.

The weapons in Teddy's war ranged from ABVD to ICE, from Adriamyin, Bleomycin, Velban, and Dacarbazine, to Ifosfamide, Cisplatin, and Etoposide. Nothing was working. Toward the end of February 2003, the ICE treatment was discontinued as there was evidence the tumors were still alive and well. With a fever of one hundred and four and fluid in his thoracic cavity, a thorocentesis was done on March 3, 2003. This relieved the pressure in his left lung and provided the doctors with more data. The fluid was tested but the results were not conclusive. A CT Scan would need to be done at Dartmouth Hitchcock. By March 6th, he learned what he already suspected. The cancer was spreading not shrinking. More decisions would need to be made. MOPP, Mechlorethamine, Vincristine, Prednisone, Procarbazine, were started on March 13th in preparation for a stem cell transplant at Dartmouth Hitchcock. The team of specialists also decided that the time had come to test Ted's siblings for a potential donor match.

Shortly after, I received a small brown package in the mail with very explicit instructions:

INSTRUCTIONS FOR DRAWING BLOOD SAMPLES FOR HLA TYPING (BONE MARROW TRANSPLANT DONOR)

1. Samples must be drawn on Monday or Tuesday only.

2. Draw 4 yellow top (ACD).

3. Label with complete name, social security number, and date. **IMPORTANT: ADD INITIALS OF PHLEBOTOMIST TO ALL TUBES. THIS IS A FEDERAL REGULATION.**

4. Repack blood tubes in inner mailing container and place box inside plastic bag. Place this inside outer box.

5. Ship by overnight Federal Express.

6. Call our laboratory to notify of sample arrival.

7. Complete the following information and send this form back with the bloods.

I read the instructions over several times and brought them with me to the lab. At 7:00 AM when I arrived at the lab, there were already a couple of people ahead of me. I could see it was going to be a busy day. A hurried assistant unlocked the door, and we blood donors searched for the sign-in clipboard. We made sure our names were at the top of the list, and then assigned ourselves to a seat in the waiting room. I grabbed a *People Magazine*, and I started to make myself comfortable, when my former high school teacher entered the room. Mr. Evan's familiar, athletic form—I'd seen him last at the gym—belied his age, but his graying temples gave it away. Rules of confidentiality and medical ethics prohibited me from asking, "Why are you here?" while I wondered why he was. I let him off the hook and told him why I was there. Mr. Evan knew Ted very well—he had him for Algebra and watched him play sports. Before he could ask me about my family, I looked into his eyes.

"Teddy has cancer and I'm here to have my blood tested to see if it might be a match, that is, if they decide to do a stem cell transplant with a donor's blood."

"I didn't know. I'm so sorry. How long has he had cancer?"

"Well, it's been diagnosed since August, but we're not sure how long he has had it."

"How did they find out?" Mr. Evan asked.

"Well, he was having trouble keeping up with his biking buddies. That was a tip that something was wrong," I answered.

"I remember when he got in that terrible accident on the basketball court," he reflected.

"I know. Everyone remembers that," I whispered.

As an out-patient, Ted was given his first treatment of MOPP. It was injected intravenously. Dutifully, Ted packed his canvas bag with extra clothes, snacks, and medications and walked the corridors of the hospital to the treatment center. Nurses greeted him and led him to his chair, where he sat, ready to be hooked to tubes.

"Did you bring some reading, Mr. Clark?"

"Nope. I have some tapes to listen to."

"I hope we don't have any trouble finding a good vein today."

"Me too," he said cringing, "that can be nasty."

Ted preferred listening to audiotapes than doing crafts. Some women are able to pass the time by knitting, sewing, and cross stitch. Although he wasn't usually one for crafts, I do remember him being pleased with a God's eye that he brought home from camp one year. Though he enjoyed reading, when he entered treatment, he never knew from day to day if he would feel up to it. Even reading could be tiresome. Watching TV became essential to keeping his sanity. Watching TV and walking were his life-line. He kept track of his exercise.

"What did you do yesterday, Mr. Clark?" The nurse asked as she prepared his arm for the IV.

"I walked a mile and a half."

"That's great. A lot of people don't do that when they're healthy. I hope you can keep it up."

Ted wasn't Brad Pitt, but his physical features were just as impressive. All my girlfriends wanted to date him and, why not? Beautiful, tanned, brown skin rippled over a muscular chest and defined biceps. Tangled, disheveled, thick blond hair turned girls' heads, but he was clueless. He had piercing Paul Newman blue eyes. His smile was a gift. Dentists drooled over his naturally straight, perfect white teeth; perfect, that is, until his fateful collision with one of his teammates during a Friday night basketball game.

I know just where I was sitting when it happened. Kathy, Brenda and I were crowded in the third row down from the top, in the left upper corner of the bleachers. I was still sweaty from my game. It was a typical, varsity high school game. I was there to cheer for Ted and the other guys.

Ted's routine consisted of one day of intravenous, seven days of pills, repeat the cycle, blood work, and then start over. In between the trips to the clinic, calls to the insurance company, and his walks, Ted took time to make Excel spread sheets. It occupied his mind. In the same way he kept track of records for Wheelabrator Technologies, he monitored the data of his cancer. One spread sheet listed his temperatures: date, time, temperature, and medication. With this information he was able to make a graph. This was how he maintained control of the situation. On another spread sheet he mapped out his "Theodore Clark to do list." (I found it interesting that he used his formal name...I never heard him refer to himself as Theodore.) On one side, he listed the items he'd completed. There were thirty-three items starting with *fixed gas grill, get gravel for driveway, change oil on car, and change oil on tractor*. The other list—"Items to do"—started with *hang gun, fixes light poles wiring, clean upstairs garage/cellar,* and ended with, *redo bathroom, re-chlorinate well, check transmission fluid in tractor and adjust clutch on tractor*. These were all things on his mind, whether he could complete them or not. What would my list look like if I was facing such uncertainty?

"Ted, Ted, he's our man...if he can't do it no one can," came to an abrupt halt! Brenda's jaw dropped and she put her hand to her mouth. I sucked in the hot, gym air. The referee blew his whistle to end the play. Kids in the crowded stands started gawking at me and asking questions.

"Did you just see what happened?"
"Isn't that your brother?"
"Do you think he'll be all right?"

"Is your mother here?"

I couldn't talk as I watched Ted's coach run to the middle of the gym. I felt sick to my stomach and my knee started to shake. My friends were well aware that Teddy Clark, with his mop of thick blond hair, and John Keely, with his tight, black curls were best friends. They scrambled for the same ball running at full speed. They reached for the ball at the exact same moment. Their bodies collided. Ted's mouth chomped down on John's skull. Ted's teeth crumbled on impact and John's skull broke apart. John collapsed and Teddy slumped to his knees. Blood splattered everywhere, staining the court floor and their white uniforms.

For weeks afterward, because Teddy wasn't able to eat solid food, he came up with a system. Anything that could be blended was pulverized and sucked down with a striped plastic straw. The swelling of his mouth caused the gooey matter to dribble down his chin. His worst concoction was a cooked hamburger, ketchup, and mashed potatoes. The red-tinged mashed potatoes with brown chunks were gross. Watching him, I couldn't stand it any longer, and asked, "Ted, how can you eat that?"

Known to have an iron stomach, he shrugged it off saying, "It all ends up in the same place anyway."

Besides walking and keeping up his spread sheets, Ted spent time with his boys. His sons enjoyed snow skiing. Corey pursued it with a passion, and picked up snow boarding—something he was good enough to compete in. That March, Ted, now half the size and form of previous years, felt strong enough to drive to Sunday River with Mom, Dad, and Kevin. Brenda and Corey had already gone ahead. It was a national competition for snow boarders. Corey was happy to have the chance to compete. Ted's jacket, two sizes too big, flapped in the breeze, and he wore his yellow baseball cap to cover his cancer-bald head. He followed his son's un-tethered form down the slope. Father and son watched grandson and son as Corey's knees buckled and straightened, buckled and straightened, buckled and straightened, simultaneously directing the rounded ski board, from one side of the course to the other. Like training the wind to blow puffs of air, Corey pushed white sprays of snow from underneath his board, creating one dazzling display after another.

"Pretty cool, huh, Dad."

"Sure is. I guess I'm too old to try that. Have you?"

"Yup. I've played around with it, but Corey really has it down."

"Lucinda." The lab technician, crossed off my name as she spoke. I turned to Mr. Evan before following her, "That was some collision, wasn't it?"

"The worst I ever saw."

"Yeah, and he still has trouble with his teeth because of it."

I took my seat in the small chair, rested my right arm on the wooden arm, and looked around the room at the cabinets, educational pamphlets, plastic bags, sterile gloves, glass tubes, and needles. I didn't linger on the needles as I handed the technician the blood donating kit. She read over the instructions.

"Who are you giving for?"

"My brother."

"What does he have?"

"Hodgkin's lymphoma."

"I've done these kits before and I'll make sure they're done right." She was respectfully soft-spoken.

"That's good to know. I guess I have to take them right to the post office after this."

"We'll seal them up properly, but get them there as soon as you can."

"I intend to go straight from here."

"I have a brother, too. Are you close?"

"Yes…we are."

She strapped the black tubing tight around my bicep and tapped the crook in my arm with her two fingers. "You have good veins." (That's what they all say.)

"Thank goodness. I'm kind of squeamish when it comes to this. If you had to poke around in there, I'm afraid I wouldn't do very well." I almost fainted giving blood for my marriage license, but that was years ago. I turned my head away from my bulging bicep and focused on the door as she reached for her needle.

Teddy helped me build good biceps. We worked out together. Instead of going to a fancy store and buying professional weights, he made his own. He found two large cans with the wrappers still on them, and filled them with cement. He found a metal rod and stuck it in the middle of the cement in one of the cans, then repeated the process after it had hardened. In a couple of days we had a set of weights. He weighed the invention. Each weighed about thirty pounds with about five pounds for the bar, to make a total of about sixty-five pounds. We used one of the long wooden benches that went with our kitchen table to lie on. Our kitchen became a weight room as we pushed the table back against the cellar wall and dragged the bench over that same 60s linoleum. The bench, free from obstructions, was placed between the table and the refrigerator. We used the blackboard to count the repetitions.

"Hey, CC, spot for me." Shirtless, barefoot, and dressed in dungarees, Teddy laid his back on the bench. One leg dropped to the left, the other to the right. He braced his knees and made himself comfortable. "Hand me the weights."

Feeling the full weight of this task I took a deep breath. I didn't want to drop them on his head. Exhaling, I grabbed the cold, metal bar and pulled the weights up to my thigh and let them rest a minute. Then, I pulled them up to my chest, careful not to bang them on my boobs (because that really hurts) and handed them to Teddy's outstretched arms. The first few lifts came easy.

He inhaled on the release and exhaled on the lift while I counted out loud, "One, two, three, four, five, six." His cheeks began to puff out on, "Seven, eight, nine, ten." He was breathing harder on, "Eleven, twelve, thirteen, fourteen." The veins in his neck were visible when we got to, "Fifteen, sixteen, seventeen." I was getting nervous and reached for the bar at eighteen, but he shook his head and pushed even harder. He wanted to get to twenty. Teddy sucked in his stomach, drew a deeper breath, then pushed up as hard as he could on nineteen shouting to me "Take it, take it" at the end of twenty. I did as I was told.

I watched as he bent at the waist and brought himself to a sitting position. Blood drained from his face. His vascular system went to work as blood re-circulated through his veins. Sweat dripped from the corners of his eyebrows. He relaxed. I walked to the blackboard that covered the distance from the kitchen door to the first set of windows. White scribbled words were sprawled across the top of the board and chalk dust covered the floor beneath the rectangular black surface—it was our family's way of communicating. Babies were announced on our blackboard, arrival and departure times of older siblings were noted on its corners. Football scores were recorded for all to see. "Happy Thanksgiving" and "Merry Christmas" were written in the nicest penmanship. (Brenda and I played hangman, and other games, on it for hours.) The blackboard served a multitude of purposes. I picked up a piece of stubby white chalk and made one long line in the middle of the board. I wrote "Teddy" at the top of one column and "Cindy" at the top of the other. I scribbled the number twenty under Teddy's name. Teddy reached up and ran his fingernails down the length of the blackboard next to his column. I shrieked—hunching my shoulders and covering my ears.

Dusting the chalk off my fingers, I walked toward the bench, "Spot for me now."

"Not yet, I want to do another set."

I had to be patient.

Ted was feeling good. Mom even said he was doing great! At the beginning of April, he drove to East Kingston with Kevin. He wanted to get some boards to make another Adirondack chair like the one he gave us for our side porch. "Finish chairs" was one of the items on his "to do" list. Pumped up on steroids, Ted was able to drive from Loudon to East Kingston. He put the brakes on in the driveway and Dad came sauntering out, before Teddy and Kevin got out of the car.

"Let's go to the barn and get the boards." Dad didn't want to hang around.

"What's the big rush, Dad?"

"I don't know. I thought you wanted to get this done."

"I do, " Teddy smirked, "just give me a minute to get out of the car, will yeah?"

"Time's a waistin'." Dad tapped his fingers on the hood of the Explorer.

"Tell me about it…" Ted dropped his head as he slowly pushed the car door open and turned to Kevin, "Kev, Kev, Grampa's on a mission, we better keep movin'."

Dad, a few steps ahead of Ted, did his best to be upbeat and think of good things to talk about. Chickens, free to roam in the yard, flapped their wings as the two approached the coop. "Shoo, shoo." Dad waved them aside. Teddy noticed a few shingles out of place on the rooftop. A trail of water separated the back yard and gushed under the bridge leading to the woods. Kevin stooped, picked up a rock, and threw it into the brook. Plunk.

"Hey, Dad, looks like your roof needs some repairs."

"I know. It's on my "to do" list."

Teddy looked back at his son, "Maybe Kevin can help you with it."

"Maybe. But, I'm not ready to tackle that project yet. How many boards do you need?"

"A few."

"Harry said we could use his planer."

"Haven't seen Uncle Harry in a while. How's he doin'?"

"Good. He's still keepin' busy aroun' the farm."

"That's good." Ted seemed glad to hear that.

My arm was beginning to get a little sore or at least uncomfortable, as the lab tech reached for the fourth tube. "They sure want a lot of blood from you."

"Let's not talk about that." I tightened and then released my fist on my lap trying to relax. I thought some more about our work-outs. Aside from the weights, there was the punching bag, but we had to leave the house to use that. Teddy hung his tan, stitched leather, store-bought punching bag from a square wooden frame on the first floor of the garage. The silver, metal hook kept the bag dangling in mid-air between beatings—it was hanging there, waiting to be abused.

Teddy tripped over the doorsill as he entered the garage. I snickered under my breath. He raised his right eyebrow but other than that, he ignored me. He walked across the cement floor, moved a bicycle, and looked for his boxing gloves. We used heavy boxing gloves, not the thinner punching bag gloves. The boxing gloves were hidden on top of the punching bag platform. He pulled one on and then the other and held both hands in front of his face, "Tie them up for me." Face to face, I was nearly the same height as Teddy. I concentrated on pulling the laces secure, but not making them too tight, "That's good," he said, "thanks."

I turned my back to Teddy and walked to the flight of stairs leading to the second floor of the garage. I took a few steps up, turned and then sat down. I bent my left knee and secured my left foot on the dirt-covered stair tread while my right leg dangled off the edge. I let it swing back and forth and back forth as Teddy grasped the punching bag between both hands.

Ba bang, ba bang, ba bang, ba bang, ba bang, ba bang, ba bang…like a drummer pounding out of control but keeping a steady beat, Teddy hit the bag with precision. Yet, every few rounds the rapid rebounding would catch him off guard. Like a tango dancer, in step with his partner, he snapped his head to the right or to the left to avoid the blow. If he didn't, he'd get hit in the face and this only made him try harder. The rhythm of the punching bag—puffy, leather gloves punching tan, leather bag, hitting wood—continued until his biceps, triceps, and wrists screamed, "Uncle." Like Luke Skywalker the force was with him. This was a kind of formal training of mind over matter for Ted. What mattered was working hard at getting in good physical condition. With fierce exercise, it didn't take long to get physically tired. It was oh so good for his mind. Besides, it was better that he use a punching bag than my arm.

Ba bang, ba bang, ba bang…like a race horse slowing his gallop, Teddy began to slow down. Ba bang, ba bang…he made one deliberate blow after another, dropping his arms after each. Ba—he hit the bag with the full force of his right arm. Bang—he hit the bag with the full force of his left arm. The bag, set free, swung back and forth and all that could be heard was the squeaking of the metal hook. Teddy's face was tomato red. Sweat covered his forehead and his arms swung to his sides, "Your turn." I helped him untie the laces and pulled off his gloves.

A warm, sweat-soaked lining enveloped my right hand as I squirmed into his glove. He helped me with the left and tied up the laces. I curled the tips of my fingers, forming a fist inside the gloves. It was hot in there. I paused and squared off in front of the bag before raising both arms. In slow motion, I began peddling my gloves across the surface of the bag. Gaining confidence, I built up speed and force until I could simulate his performance. Hitting the bag as fast as I could, and getting cocky, I miscalculated—the bag whacked me in the cheek. I felt the sting of the bag's stitches as my upper lip began to swell. Snot ran from my right nostril. I wiped it away with the back of his glove.

"Goin' a little too fast?" Teddy chuckled, as I came after him with a swing at his shoulder. He deflected the punch, grabbed my arm, and swung me around backward. In seconds, he had me in a half nelson, forcing me to bend over. My long, straight brown hair covered my eyes on both sides of my face, but I could see his sneakers. I stomped on his big toe. It startled him but he came back even stronger, wrapping both arms around my waist and wrestling me to the floor. I struggled and elbowed him in his side. He got me in a scissor hold and squeezed my belly tight enough to suck out all my air. "You give?" Not able to breathe, I could only nod my head.

He lifted his leg on top of me off and pulled out his other leg from under me. Having cashed in my last ounce of energy, I let my legs and arms collapse on the dirty, cold, cement floor while Teddy pushed away. Then, like making angels in the snow, I began to move again, sweeping sawdust with all four limbs. I could feel the wet puddles of sweat that had collected under both armpits. The rush of adrenaline, the rapid heart beating, the roughness of physical contact, the ridiculousness of me fighting him was exhilarating. We worked it out—believe it or not, this was fun stuff.

"I've filled all the tubes. You're good to go."

"Thanks. You did a nice job."

"Good luck with your brother."

"Thanks."

By the middle of April Teddy's fevers were back. This was a strong indication that MOPP wasn't working. Nothing could stop his cancer. Ted also learned that none of his sisters or his brother was a perfect match. The doctors decided to get blood samples from Brenda, Corey, and Kevin. BEACOPP was started. The acronym stood for Bleomycin, Etoposide, Doxorubicin, Cyclophosphamide, Vincristine, Procarbazine, and Prednisone. It was another trial combination of drugs—another form of chemotherapy. The sounds of those drugs made me think they would be strong enough to kill my brother—not cure him. More tests, PET scan, CT scan, and a bone marrow biopsy were done on April 11th. Ted was admitted to Dartmouth Hitchcock.

When Pat, Dave, Muffy and I arrived to visit him on April 12th, we were greeted with more bad news. A nurse, visibly alarmed, met us in the hall.

"Ted's blood pressure has dropped. We're moving him to intensive care. We'll come talk to you when we have him stable." Just then, a still-alive body, covered with white sheets, was wheeled by us on a stretcher. The gurney was moving fast and it carried our brother. We stood to the side and held our breath, not prepared to see him in this condition. We found our way to the waiting room. Other concerned family members of other sick patients were slumped in comfortable chairs, talking in hushed tones. I turned to Pat and asked, "Did you see how white he was?"

"He's in rough shape, but he's going to make it. He's a tough guy. I don't know anyone tougher than Ted."

I knew Pat meant what he said. Somehow, this was comforting.

Many times Pat had told me the story of Teddy—or "Boris," as he was nicknamed—and the guys in the high school Audio-Visual club. Sneaking by the "AV" inner sanctum, at the top of the stairs in the new science building, gave me the creeps. God forbid I was ever asked to go there to get some audio visual equipment for one of my teachers. There was so much testosterone oozing from the pores of the cramped room (where the football players hung out) that it seeped into the hall and made me lose control of my senses. I was an underclass female—

distinctly different than the occupants of "that room." Crass remarks cackled across the corners of the room about passing female forms, "Look at the tits on her." Rambunctious laughter erupted on cue. I avoided going by the door, never mind poking my head in (so did Kathy and Brenda) whenever possible.

It didn't surprise me that outrageous acts of subhuman behavior may occur behind the closed door of the AV club—I didn't really want to know about them. Yet, Pat told me a story about Ted that left an impression. Teddy, unfortunately, could be the brunt of jokes. He used to mix up his words. One time when we double-dated, he asked for walnut "sludge" instead of walnut fudge. Ted and his date, and Pat and I, laughed about it the rest of the night. On another double-date, we were eating at a Chinese restaurant and he dipped his egg roll into his date's tea instead of into the dipping sauce. Teddy made smudge marks on anything he touched. Once, he accidentally put his elbow in my homemade lemon meringue pie. He was forever skipping a button in his shirt leaving one shirt tail longer than the other. There were lots of reasons the guys poked fun at him. What frustrated Pat was that this one bully, a long time member of the AV club, mercilessly teased the hell out of Teddy who sat back and took it. Pat would say, "Teddy, you're so much stronger; you could beat the shit out of that guy. I don't understand why you let him get away with that crap." Teddy would shrug his shoulders and say, "It's not worth it."

Teddy wasn't ready to go yet. That night he fought the fevers, the diarrhea, and the effects of seven strong chemotherapy drugs. By morning his blood pressure was stable. Pat and I slipped into his hospital room, as if parents of a newborn, and tiptoed to the side of his bed. His eyes were closed and he was breathing. This is something parents look for. I mouthed, "Let's not wake him up." We turned back around and left without disturbing him, wondering if he felt our presence as we snuck in and out of his room. I wondered how many others would have to do the same over the course of his hospital stay. It was unsettling to watch a grown man sleep, but not like a baby.

A steady stream of visitors—his wife, children, mother, father, cousins, brother, sisters, nieces, nephews, and friends—continued to flow in and out of the hospital. All reported back to one another on his status. Again, each conversation was an intrusion into a private person's life. It was hard not to be intrusive when we were all so concerned. Some visitors made him laugh, some made him cry, some walked with him, some watched movies with him, but we all came and each of us made a difference. It was hard for all of us to see his bottom lip quiver and know that he was unable to say what was on his mind. We were not mind readers and could only guess. Becky, my oldest sister, asked, "Would you like me to rub your feet?" (She was one of three nurses in our family—my mom, my daughter, and her.) Ted's unexpected response was, "Yes. That would be good."

I watched as Becky tugged at the sheets at the bottom of his bed to uncover his swollen feet. She pulled the sock off of one foot and filled the palm of her right hand with baby lotion. She bent over his bare foot and began massaging his heel, then gently moved up to the arch of his foot.

"How did you sleep last night?" Becky asked.

"Not great. I've been watching the History Channel; at least there are some pretty good shows on that. You'd be surprised at what comes on late at night." Ted tried to be optimistic.

"How's your appetite?"

"It's all right, but it gets pretty boring. They won't let me eat anything good." Watching Becky, I thought to myself—if he lets her do this, maybe he'll let me.

The warm touch of Becky's hands made Ted relax. For the moment, he could abandon his "tough guy" exterior.

Savored homemade spaghetti smell met me at the door. It made me put down my guard—I had had a miserable day. The "D" I got on my geometry exam floated out the window, along with the penetrating aroma of slow-cooking, tomatoes, garlic, and oregano. It was as soothing as a gentle foot massage. I glanced at the blackboard and saw, "Happy Birthday Ted!" Mom was making Aunt Eleanor's coveted recipe, the one she brought with her from Austria. Aunt Eleanor escaped the war with my Uncle Paul. My Aunt Eleanor carried this recipe along with all her memories. It didn't come in the one, small leather trunk she brought with her to America. Yet, it did come across the Atlantic Ocean and found its way to our home. Something that travels that far has to be steeped in love. Same as in the book *Like Water for Chocolate*, the cooks, as well as those who eat the cooking, are zapped with a heightened pleasure that cannot be explained. It can only be experienced. Teddy's favorite birthday meal was also mine.

"When Becky gets done rubbing your feet would you like to go for a walk?" I asked from the foot of Ted's bed.

"Sure." Ted did not hesitate.

The scenery was different than that of the outdoors. Narrow corridors were lined with patient rooms, doctors, and nurses, but somehow the walk was still therapeutic. After Becky had thoroughly massaged his feet and pulled his socks back on, I looked for his sneakers. I found them under his bed and holding one in my hand, wondered what to do next. "I can get them on," he let me know.

With Becky ready to reach out and grab one elbow and me the other, we escorted Ted by the first nurses' station. His loose-fitting sweat pants fell limp around his ankles. He took baby steps and smiled up at one of the nurses, "These are two of my sisters. You know, I have five."

She smiled back, "I know, Teddy. You told me all about them. Which ones are these?"

"This one's Becky. She's the nurse, so you better not mess with her. And this one's Cindy...I mean Lucinda. Now that she's grown up she likes to go by that name." I rolled my eyes but let him continue. "They're here to help me with my exercise today."

"You need help, Ted." She was joking with him, "You've been lying around too much lately. You need to get out of that room." Then she added, "Having five sisters must have been pretty rough on you."

"Not too bad." He turned his attention to the floor and continued walking. He concentrated on taking the corner at the end of the corridor. We tried not to bump into each other as we walked down the next corridor, made the next corner, and then made it back. He looked up and counted out loud at the nurses' station, "one."

The same nurse looked at us, "How many are you going for today, Ted?"

"Maybe five. It depends if my sisters can keep up with me."

"Maybe this would be a good time for me to put you in a half nelson." I smiled at the nurse.

Even when I thought I could "take him," I couldn't. It was my sixteenth birthday and we just finished a game of "horse." I caught Teddy glaring at me from the corner of his eye. I knew I was in trouble. He warned me in the morning that I was due for sixteen spankings. I could still remember the burning sensation on my butt from last year. I saw his quick feet darting in my direction and heard him warn, "I'm gonna getcha."

I threw the basketball up in the air, hoping it would trip him up, and then took off as fast as I could. I ran in back of the barn and sprinted for the pear tree. Starting to laugh while taking a quick look behind me, I saw the empty space between us disappearing. I tried to use his "zig zag" maneuver on him. I ran in a straight line from the pear tear to the trash barrel and then made a quick turn toward the clothesline. My dodge to the left was meant to throw him off, but you can't beat a trickster with his own trick. It only delayed the inevitable. Teddy captured me as I grabbed the pole, holding up the clothesline, and tried to spin away. Instead of escaping, Teddy spun me around and I landed on a pile of freshly mown grass. The short, green clippings tickled the tip of my nose, but I couldn't scratch because Teddy had my hands pinned under me. With his left knee on my back he raised his right arm and began spanking. Whack! His hand slapped my butt and made me squirm but the "pinch to grow an inch" made me scream. Mission accomplished, he stood up, "Happy birthday, CC."

    The thumb and fingerprint bruise where he pinched me lasted weeks. (I always did bruise easily.) It finally faded from a deep purple and blue to a muted yellow and orange. As I spit strands of hair out of my mouth, I looked up from the ground, "Thanks, Ted. I'll get you back for this."

    On April 26th Ted had his stem cells harvested. The doctors took as many stem cells out of his blood as they possibly could. Those stem cells would be treated to remove any cancer and then be put back into him to rejuvenate his blood system. That night, we prayed they collected a sufficient amount. If they did, Ted could go home for a couple of days before returning for the stem cell transplant procedure, which would require him to stay four to six weeks in isolation. He had already been in the hospital for a couple weeks and the doctors wanted him to spend some quality time in familiar surroundings with his wife and sons, before the final stage of treatment. The space between the four walls of his hospital room, and between us, was beginning to close in. I thought about him constantly. Ted remained dedicated to his stationary bike and he continued to walk the wing of the Cancer Center, but there was no "zig zagging" his way out of this.

    The next day, as we sat at her kitchen table, Mom filled me in, "We had a whole bunch of calls today back and forth about Ted. In the morning, they told Ted they were going to have to try to get some more stem cells removed. Then, later in the day, they got a second report that contradicted the first one. Eventually, the doctors determined that they did have enough cells and Ted could go home." Mom's voice grew weaker as she told me the story of the day's events. By the time she got to, "Brenda went and got him and he called me from home," she was beginning to cry. I could barely hear her words, as she bowed her head, and ended with, "I'm so glad he got to go home."

Yours is not to Question Why... Yours is just to Do or Die

Email is a marvelous intervention. It helped our family keep in touch about Ted, and it was efficient. I often wonder what it would have been like without this means of communication. Mom and Dad tried to keep the six of us, and our families, informed of any changes with Ted. It's overwhelming to think of the number of calls we would have had to make. As it was, we still needed to rely on phone calls some of the time. But, by using email, updates on Ted's condition could get circulated with a click of the mouse. The information could be detailed, informative, lengthy, or short, funny or sad, but it was there for everyone to see. News could be quickly shared. I opened my email to the following note from my younger brother.

From: Jim Clark
To: The Clarks
Sent: Wednesday, April 30, 2003 8:49 PM
Subject: ted's day 4/30/03

Hello Everyone,
Just spoke to Ted and he had a long day at Hanover today. He had 5 tests blood, ekg, pulmonary etc. His WBC count high, and his RBC is a little low. He has a sufficient number of stem cells that had allowed him to come home on Sunday. The doctors told him they thought he would have to undergo a bone marrow transplant and did not think he would do so well at getting enough stem cells. This was another good surprise. (He didn't have to undergo a bone marrow transplant.)
Sat. 5/3 he has to go back to Hanover at 12:00 to have a Cat Scan. The plan is to start his next chemo on Tuesday 5/6. He will be on this regiment for 5 straight days, have a couple days off and then have his stem cells put back. We then just have to wait and see how he does.

As part of this regiment he is also going to sign a consent form (case study) for a new drug which is to help stimulate his immune system.

Thursday and Friday this week should be light and he will only have to give himself Lominx shots for blood thinning, and have a visiting nurse come to keep his port clean.

Jim

I don't think Jim slept well that night. In fact, he probably tossed and turned until he got up and took some Tylenol PM. He might have gone on the computer and started doing more endless research about Hodgkin's lymphoma. Or, he might have looked over the information he got from his doctor friend about stem cell transplants. Or, he might have started making lists for work the next day, or... he could have taken his bike out of his cellar and ridden it into the woods—like his brother was known to do.

At odd hours of the night, Ted straddled his bike, called for his dog, Jesse, and took off into the woods. Folklore is filled with legends of local, every day people committing oddly eccentric acts. I remember Midnight Palmer knocking on our door late at night to sell his vegetables. He used to walk the streets of Kingston with a push cart after most people had gone to bed. A local veterinarian, by the name of Doc Treadwell, has been sighted galloping through the shadows of serene moonlit evenings. And, Ted's nighttime romps through the woods caused packs of coyotes to wake up his neighbors.

A big man with a big horse spotted at 1:00 in the morning is something to talk about. I don't think Doc Treadwell cared about that. In the same way, I don't think Teddy cared what anyone else thought about him wearing a flashlight atop his head to guide him over the trails in back of his Loudon home, and drift where the spirit moved him at random hours of late evenings. Years from now his friends will say, "Remember when Ted Clark used to take his dog, Jesse, and ride his bike through the woods at night. What a guy."

During intermission—the nine days between Ted being home and returning to Dartmouth Hitchcock—life in our family went on. Ted's sons, Corey and Kevin, both excelled in track meets that Ted was able to attend. Brenda ran. And, Teddy walked. Mom worked on her painting of a marsh scene. Jim's son, Jordan, was Peter Pan in his class play. Brenda ran. And, Teddy walked. Another nephew, Scottie, played in an AAU basketball tournament at UNH. A grandchild, Brynna Ashton Edmiston, was baptized. My granddaughter, Kaylie Jessica

Marcoux, was born. Mom recorded all of these events in her diary, along with and beside the information about Ted. The tapestry of our family life was being woven with surprising bits of joy against a backdrop of troubling thoughts of Ted. Throughout it all, Brenda ran. And, Teddy walked.

Ted's love of nature, of trees, of wilderness, prompted him and Brenda to purchase land in Franconia, New Hampshire in 1994. In Franconia, he worked as a dairy inspector and first met his friend Jay. He also started dating Brenda. Jay told us all about his "wild trips" with Teddy, "racing and trying to push each other over…on x-country skis down the Mount Washington auto road from timberline." For Ted, an opportunity to explore the White Mountains, with skis, snow shoes, hiking boots, or on a bike, was ample reason to push the limits. The Kangamangus River, running through the White Mountains, presented a challenge. He plunged into the icy, rushing water in early spring. So what if there were pointed rocks jutting out from beneath the surface. So what if the sign at the top of Mount Adams warned, "Danger. Turn back," just like the one the Cowardly Lion came upon, in the dark forest of *The Wizard of Oz*. Challenges like these were Ted's green light. So what if he was getting blisters from hiking all day, he'd take care of that later. These obstacles were meant to be ignored, not taken seriously.

Ted was frugal. He didn't even take out a mortgage when he built his house. Yet, he could not pass up the chance to buy an expansive, seventy-one acre, piece of land abutting Cannon Mountain. His property was acre upon unsettled acre, left to be explored, selectively cut, and maintained for outdoor enjoyment. The land was something for him and his family to hang on to for the future. I can only imagine what he thought about as he silently surveyed his "saving for retirement land" two days before he was admitted back to Dartmouth Hitchcock Hospital—another very different place nestled among tall New Hampshire trees.

It would be presumptuous to think that I could know what was on his mind that day, but I do know his steps were slow and he was thoughtful. With his life in limbo his stamina—both mental and physical—was being pushed to the limits. He couldn't chase his son through the woods. He could barely walk. As Ted's world was beginning to crumble around him, Mom made an entry in her diary about "The Old Man of the Mountain." The sharp features of a forehead, nose and chin could be viewed one thousand, two hundred feet above Profile Lake. This "stone face" was one of New Hampshire's most famous tourist attractions and captured the attention of everyone who saw it—"The Old Man of the Mountain" could be seen from I-93 in Franconia Notch State Park. Some people merely caught a glimpse of him from the highway as they were driving by, others died trying to climb his rocky surface. On May 4, 2003, people in New Hampshire woke up to discover that this famous granite profile was gone. I think it's ironic. At the very time that Ted was falling apart, "The Old Man of the Mountain" disappeared from the face of the mountain. Ted's physical profile would soon be gone as well.

Subject: First day of chemo
From: Clark, Ted-J
Date: Thu, 8 May 2003

Hi gang
Yesterday I survived the first round of chemo...it reminded me of my college days...where you promise yourself that you will never have too much to drink again.
The chemo drugs (BCNU) are suspended and preserved in alcohol, so not only do you have the effects of the chemo drugs, you get the added bonus of straight injection of alcohol. The first day of chemo is supposed to be the worst, and now I have that behind me.
Today I'm doing much better my stomach and head are settling down and I was able to ride the stationary bike for a half hour.

Thirty eight thousand, eight hundred and eighty minutes! How do you measure a month in the hospital? In blood work? In temperature? In blood pressure? In a sunset? In a sunrise? The constant checking of body functions was measured moment by moment. Ted was fortunate to have a room with a view to the outside, and it was on the first floor. There wasn't much to see by most people's standards. Ted was lucky to see out, even though his world was diminished. He could observe visitors coming and going, the wind blowing leaves up in the air on windy days, and the cascading degrees of light over dark and dark over light.

The author, M. Scott Peck, wrote *A Bed by the Window* in which he describes how in nursing homes the coveted bed is the one by the window. Yet, in order to get that bed by the window, someone has to die. Teddy had a bed by the window. Perhaps there were nights, like when we were children sharing the same bedroom, when he was afraid of what lurked beyond that window.

Ted had the top bunk, I had the bottom. Sometimes that would change, depending on whether he woke up from a bad dream. For some reason unknown to me, Teddy was plagued by the fear of lions getting loose, jumping through the window, and leaping onto his bed. On occasion, I remember waking in the morning to discover that he had dragged his sleeping bag out in the middle of the night and fallen asleep on the floor outside Mom and Dad's bedroom. On other restless nights, he woke me up with gentle prodding, "Cindy, Cindy, get up and switch beds with me." Half asleep and totally unaware of what was happening, I would mumble, "What for?" Softly, breathing on my face, he whispered, "Because if the lions get loose, they might jump through the window and up onto my bed." If I was more awake, I might have been able to reason with him: "Why is it better for me to switch to the top bunk and get attacked by the lions?" But I didn't because, as he would later say to me, "Yours is not to question why…yours is just to do or die."

Subject: Hi Gang
From: Clark, Ted-J
Date: Wed. 14 May 2003

Hi gang
Well, today was rest day………………………………….. my last day of chemo was yesterday. Also today I had enough Cat Scan and chest x-ray, I haven't seen the result yet, but Dr. said I was doing very good. I have my fingers crossed that this chemo treatment has done its job.
Tomorrow the doctors are planning to put my frozen stem cells back into my bone marrow and jump start the immune system and getting all the system working. It probably will be another couple of weeks to see how well the new stem cells are working.

It was spring. It was time for Pat and me to get the camps ready for another season at Lake Fairlee in Post Mills, Vermont. This meant getting up early on Saturday morning, driving two and a half hours to Vermont, working on the camps all day, sleeping in the Honeymoon Cottage, and visiting Ted on Sunday on our way home. This became our routine.

Like Morgaine, high priestess in *The Mists of Avalon*, searching for a way to separate the mist, I felt the power of the lake. It brought me to another world. Dawn, weighted down with a damp fog, gave me respite from the real work world. "What a world, what a world, what a world." A bright morning sun usually startled me into its existence. I much preferred a slow-moving, moist mist to bring me to my senses. There was a list of chores to be done but it could wait.

I awoke in the blue painted, metal bed and listened to the water gently massaging the rocks imbedded in the shoreline. Peeling away three layers of heavy blankets—I braced myself for the rush of cool air and reached for my clothes. I flinched as my feet touched the floor. I pulled on my purple, green, orange, and black striped pair of 80s "jams" and purple sweater, and found my socks. This "get up" may have scared my neighbors back home, but in Post Mills, Vermont I really blended. Sneaking with my "camp only" sneakers in one hand, I fingered the pull-out couch with the other, trying not to stub my toe on my way through the living room and out to the porch.

The porch, screened on two sides facing the lake, was wrapped in Mother Earth's packaging. I was by myself inside this wonderful package. I didn't care how long it took to get unwrapped. Water, air, and fog were everywhere. I pulled out the ice cream parlor wooden chair and sat at the kitchen table that was covered with a green and white checked plastic tablecloth. Bending to lace my sneakers, I took note of the peeling, red paint that forever needed repair. I straightened up and searched my surroundings for familiar markings. To my right was a tall pine tree where I once observed a blue heron perched on a thick root at its base. I watched that heron for about fifteen minutes before it flew off. To my left was a small cove where our children swung from a rope strung from a tree way up the rocky ledge. My nephew Joey broke his wrist falling down that embankment when the branch broke. His wrist hurt, and it was bad—but it didn't hurt badly. It wasn't as bad as the time my son Matt hooked him in the forehead with his fishhook. (That ruined our Fourth of July.) In front of me was the lake, but I couldn't see to the other side where I knew there was a bridge.

Dave, my sister Muffy's husband, was a faithful visitor to Dartmouth Hitchcock. He could say things that others wouldn't dare to say. Dave has a way about him. His brand of teasing is generally taken in stride. (He is known to get on a theme.) Although Ted and Dave may not have had the closest relationship, they knew each other well enough that Dave was free to be himself. And, it was fine with Teddy. While Ted struggled for weeks with nausea, chills, and diarrhea, Dave provided comic relief, and daily visits to check on his progress. Dave didn't hold back.

"Did you shit in your pants today?"

"Yeah, Dave. You should've been here. You could have helped the nurses clean me up."

"I'm good. But, I'm not that good. What color was your puke?"

"Kinda reddish."

"You gotta knock off that fruity Gatorade and switch to the orange."

"Yeah, Dave. I'll get right to it. I'm here for your entertainment."

"What movie do you want to watch tonight?"

"How about *Night of the Living Dead*?"

"Sorry. Blockbuster is all out of that one. How about *Return of the Living Dead*?"

"Go for it. If they don't have that you can always pick up *Live and Let Die*."

"Sure, Ted. But wouldn't you rather see a *Pink Panther* movie?"

"Yeah, yeah…why don't you make yourself useful and hand me 'the phun'." Ted was good at mimicking Peter Sellers as inspector Clouseau.

Dave handed him the phone and turned to leave the room, allowing him privacy, "I'll be back."

As he walked down the hospital corridor Dave made a note to himself to check with Ted's doctor. He was very concerned about Ted's chills, weight loss, white blood counts, and continued nausea. It didn't take Dr. Bates long to get back to him.

Dr. Bates assured Dave that Ted was making progress. Because Ted was so heavily treated prior to getting his transplant, it could be a reason that the engraftment period may take longer. Dr. Bates suspected his chills were likely caused by some of the antifungal medications Ted was getting. Weight loss was expected. He hoped as Ted's body engrafted, things would settle down. And, after the doctors were able to stop most of the medications, the nausea, the weight loss, and the chills should get better.

I took my thirty-five millimeter camera from the fireplace mantle, and left the Honeymoon Cottage, careful not to let the screen door slam. With hot air balloons rising at any time, and wildlife roaming unexpectedly from out of the woods, there was always a need for a camera. I tried to have my camera with me at all times.

Treacherous roots spread from the cottage to the dock. I hung my camera around my neck and navigated across the dirt and pine needles, and down the slope to the wooden planks that carried me safely to water's edge. I stepped over abandoned swim goggles. At the end of the dock I inhaled, casting my eyes toward Camp Billings—blanketed by a light layer of hazy fog. In the distance, I could hear scraping of oars against oar locks as a row boat made a path through the water. This was the only sound I could hear. A shiver ran up my spine as I exhaled a breath of air. Like a smoker, I tipped my head back and watched my breath float from my mouth. As my breath faded, I was eager to take another drag.

Between the surface of the water and the cloudlike veil, I watched the lone row boat emerge, coming closer and closer toward me. A father was rowing the boat, while his son stood at the bow with his hands tightly holding his fishing pole. I took my camera off my neck and flipped off the lens cover. I lifted it up to my eyes and brought the scene into focus. The man and the boy were silhouetted figures frozen in dew time, as the lake wrapped its misty tentacles around them. I snapped the picture.

I was so engrossed in watching the two fishermen that I did not hear Pat approach from behind. I felt his hand on my shoulder.

"Mornin'. Whatcha thinkin' about?"

"Ted."

"Me, too. I think about him a lot. More than you know."

"When did you wake up?"

"Soon after you left. I just laid there."

"Teddy wouldn't be fishing, would he?"

"No. It wasn't like him."

From June 2nd to June 7th, Ted remained confined to a hospital room. A huge, white board registered his daily counts. From his bed, it was easy for him to read the numbers. Headings at the top read: WBC, RBC, and ANC. He was—and so were we—particularly concerned with the ANC report, as that indicated how many new cells were being generated. This was the first thing that visitors looked at. It was also the way Teddy kept track of his progress, or lack thereof.

On Monday, Teddy had a fever of 102.2. Cold cloths were placed on his head to cool him down. Mom was able to give him a foot massage and read to him. She read him family tales about the farm that had been written by one of his cousins. On Tuesday, his counts started to rise. Brenda still couldn't come in to see him because of her cold. She had to talk to him with a walkie-talkie through his window. On Wednesday, a physical therapist started to work with him on strengthening exercises. His WBC and ANC were going up. He hadn't had a fever in over thirty-six hours. On Thursday, Muffy got to see that he was improving. Friday, he was much better. Saturday, he had another transfusion. Sunday, we visited.

Before entering Ted's room, we had to wash our hands. Outside his room were anti-bacterial soap, a wash sink, and paper towels. Everyone had to use them. My previous "Infection Control" training came in handy. I learned one way to ensure you have washed an adequate amount of time, is to sing 'Happy Birthday," while vigorously rubbing. Both palms and backs of your hands should be properly scrubbed. I held my hands under running water and sang to myself, "Happy birthday to you, happy birthday to you, happy birthday dear Teddy, happy birthday to you."

As usual, he was sitting up in bed looking over his menu. He smiled when we entered his space. I wanted to give him a great big hug but precautions prohibited me from getting too close to his face. I slid alongside his IV pole and touched his arm, "How are you?" It was obvious he wasn't well. He had no hair, pale color, and dry, cool skin. If he wasn't having a fever, he was often cold. Sometimes, he shook uncontrollably. He gave his standard reply, "So so. What have you guys been up to?" He did seem to enjoy hearing what other people were doing. I tried to think of things to tell him that might be interesting, before I got to his room.

"Well, besides working on the camps, we went out to dinner on Friday night to celebrate Becky and Ron's thirty-fifth anniversary."

"Oh really, has it been that long? When was their anniversary anyway?" It was a given that Teddy didn't keep track of events like anniversaries. Sometimes, he forgot his own.

"June 6th."

"Where did you go out to eat?" Ted always enjoyed a good meal. His thoughts lately tended more and more toward food. The more he was deprived of something juicy to eat, the more he wanted it.

"Becky and Ron made reservations at the Exeter Inn for Mom, Dad, Pat and me. That's where their reception was. They wanted to revisit the Inn. You know Becky and Ron, they're not usually ones for fancy restaurants but this was a pretty special occasion."

"I guess so. What did you have to eat?"

"Becky and I had salmon. You know Dad, he had scallops," I couldn't bring myself to describe the meal in greater detail and quickly changed the subject, "The waitress thought it was pretty cool that we were together celebrating this wedding anniversary and that it had been such a long time since Becky and Ron had eaten there. There was a lot of reminiscing goin' on. We talked about how you almost missed their wedding."

It was prematurely ninety degrees on Saturday, June 6, 1968 and Teddy had to go to "the island." Mom probably wanted him to stick around the house, but he probably snuck off when she was busy with other wedding preparations. "The island," located in the middle of Kingston Lake, was owned by an uncle. It was where we all learned to water ski and where we all wanted to be in the summer. Teddy jumped on his bike, rode it in back of the garage, ran to where the boat was docked and jumped in. He pulled the motor on his red hydroplane, and raced across the lake past Kingston State Park to the island. He escaped.

The wedding was at 6:00 in the evening. As the hour drew closer and closer, Teddy was nowhere to be seen. The flurry of a bride, the maid-of-honor, mother-of-the-bride, three bridesmaids, a flower girl, and other related family members frantically getting ready for a wedding, was enough to make any fourteen-year-old boy want to run away. Run away, run away, run away.

In the midst of the confusion someone asked, "Where's Teddy?"

Someone answered, "He's gone to the island."

Mom said, "I hope he gets back in time."

I thought, "He's in trouble now."

A drive from our house to Kingston Congregational Church would take approximately ten minutes. By 5:00 PM, I was dressed in a long white dress with a royal blue top. Someone must have curled my hair. I wore girly, flat, white shoes. Attached to my back was a full length, royal blue train fastened to my dress with Coast Guard buttons. Becky was marrying an officer in the Coast Guard. We each carried one red rose down the aisle. This was a military red, white, and blue wedding. The night before, Becky and Ron rehearsed marching under the arch of swords held high by handsome Coast Guard groomsmen. I was twelve and was escorted by "Peaches," Ron's best friend and fellow officer.

I was in my bedroom fiddling with my white gloves, trying to figure out how I was going to wear them. I had a vicious case of purulent, pustulant, inflamed poison ivy. The itchy line of bubbles ran up and down the sides of my pinky and middle fingers of my right hand. It was uncomfortable to put my gloves on. I heard Mom put her foot down in the kitchen, "Teddy still isn't back yet. We may have to leave without him." She was furious. It was too bad because this was her first daughter's wedding day! The best made plans were quickly disappearing.

Debbie, daughter number two, was dressed the same as me. She wore slightly higher shoes than me, and raised the hem of her dress as she stepped from the porch. She looked across The Plains and saw a boy on his bike. She yelled as loud as she could, "Hurry up; we're getting ready to leave." Teddy stood on the pedals and picked up speed, wet hair plastered to his forehead. He spun across the side road and into our yard, leaning his bike against the garage. "Quick, take a shower and I'll wait for you." Debbie would have to drive him separately. She paced back and forth, and rearranged her hair piece several times, until Teddy banged his elbow on the bathroom door and staggered out. Teddy never could *clean up good*. When he arrived at the church, his hair was still wet—a tuft of matted snarls visible from the back.

Teddy remembered the event but wasn't feeling guilty, "So, what was the big deal about that? I made it to the church on time."

"Yeah, you did, Ted, but Mom sure had a fit," I replied.

"Ah, people make such a fuss over those things." Ted was still defending his actions, but he did have a bit of a grin.

"I'm surprised you made it to your own wedding on time. And, that you had it in a church. How did Brenda manage that?" I wanted to know.

"I don't know." Ted didn't offer any explanation.
I glanced at Pat, "It was Muffy that almost messed up our wedding."

"Oh, what did she do?" Teddy asked.

"She decided to pick flowers for our wedding decorations and ended up at the beach. Guess she lost track of time, too. It was another hot one. Mom wasn't sweating just because of the heat," I explained.
"It figures. Mom's always been such a worrier," Ted qualified.

I looked back at Ted, "Pat and Dave almost made us late for your wedding."

"Really. Why is that?" Teddy looked at Pat.

"You tell him, Pat," I urged Pat to answer.

Pat took over from here, "It was a play-off game during "March Madness." North Carolina was playing against Georgetown. We were in the hotel room watching Michael Jordon and Patrick Ewing duke it out. It was a wicked good game. Dave and I wanted to see the end but Muffy and Cindy made us leave before it was over."

"Gee. I'm sorry about that." Ted was grinning.

"No big deal, Boris. We just missed an ending to a really good game. Just the sacrifices you have to make for a good buddy."

I watched as nature uncovered Lake Fairlee, moment by moment, and more of the opposite shore came into view. It was like Mom gently pulling away a soft blue blanket from her sleeping baby boy—ever so carefully so as not to wake him up, yet completely so that an eager visitor could see him. As Camp Billings awakened, Pat and I walked from the dock and started up the hill toward the Crow's Nest. We needed to figure out our day. I noticed the gully running down the hill was deeper than last weekend, due to a heavy rain storm. Pat would want to throw some dirt into that. Tree branches, also knocked down from the storm, were blocking the driveway.

"I want to cut that tree down." Pat had his eye on the pine, closest to the Crow's Nest. "The only one I would trust to help me with it is Ted."

We stood in the driveway, looking at the clean lines of the brown boards, covering the camp. It was in remarkable contrast to the old, moldy, tar shingles. "Boris had a blast tearing down the old Crow's Nest…"

I held my camera tight to my chest and prepared to record this "day of reckoning." The first picture I took was of Ted. He didn't wait around for instructions. There was work to be done. He grabbed a pick ax, carried it up on the roof over the kitchen, and started ripping up shingles. The picture reflects an energetic man in his 40s, bent at the waist, unshaven, with his tangle of sun-blonde hair flopping over his ears. Jimmy watched him for a minute before joining him. As if they were children crushing a sandcastle, Teddy and Jimmy were determined to smash this building to pieces. Shingles, loose boards, and heavy, long strings of electrical wires started flying into the air. They landed in chaos in the big, green, Waste Management dumpster we rented for the weekend. It was a huge, empty dumpster but by the end of the day, it was overflowing.

I tried to get them to stop for lunch but they wouldn't. Too much testosterone was flowing for this tactical assignment. It bothered them that they had to break long enough to figure out how to cut down the supporting beams of the living room. Midway through the day, I took a picture of Pat, Ted, and Jim standing in the middle of a barren living room, windows knocked out, wearing work gloves and safety goggles. They discussed how they should saw through the roof.

"We can cut through there." Ted was sure it was okay.

"I'm not so sure. Let's think about it." Pat wanted to do it right.

"Why not just hack through that one?" Jim pointed to a beam by the fireplace.

After a brief period of "hemmin' and hawin'," they agreed on a plan, and fired up their saws. Once again, I made my way out of the immediate vicinity, and prayed that no one would get hurt. They successfully sawed through wood and shingles, and prepared the Crow's Nest for demolition. With all major supports torn apart, all windows and doors gone, and the building ready for collapse, they devised the finishing touch.

I climbed down the steep, brush-covered ledge in back of the Crow's Nest and stood as far back as I could, but close enough to get a few final shots. I looked up from below and watched Pat tie a massive, yellow rope around the corner of the kitchen's remaining beam near the roof. As if playing a one-sided game of tug-of-war, the guys lined up on the edge of the cliff and pulled, and pulled, and pulled. It wasn't for forty days and forty nights, but Conan the barbarian would be proud. The Crow's Nest fell apart as boards crashed to the ground and a plume of dust flew above the collapsed building. Teddy, with his white t-shirt poking out from under his faded, sawdust covered sweatshirt, stood back with his hands on his hips appreciating the wreckage. That was a picture, too.

"So, when do you think you'll be able to come home?" I wanted to know the answer before we left.

"My counts seem to be going up. I might be able to get home this week."

"Wow, Ted. That would be great."

"It sure will."

"Is there anything we can get you?"

"A great big juicy steak would be nice."

"You got it, just as soon as you're given the green light. We have to get goin' now." Pat and I slunk toward the door.

"Thanks for comin' in."

"We wish we could do more."

Pat and I walked the long corridor from Ted's room to the exit's automatic doors. People were coming and going. From the outside of the hospital, down the sidewalk, to the parking lot, we didn't say a word. We reached Pat's black Ford Explorer, unlocked the doors, and climbed in. I buckled my seatbelt, hunched over and burst into tears.

Home at Last

"Ted's at home!" Mom was elated. This time, the good news spread through the family phone tree on June 10, 2003. There was no pomp and circumstance as Ted gathered his meager belongings from room one hundred twenty five. A hospital attendant wheeled him to his car. Young, beautiful, caring women—like my daughter—with RN next to their names, had shared moments of intimacy, meant to be private with Teddy. These angels came to Ted in the dead of night. The nights that we could only imagine what pain he was suffering, they were there with him. They came to wish him well. They wanted to see him live. He was one of their favorite patients. Or, so they said. Perhaps, they said that about all their patients, or perhaps, he really was special to them. One of the nurses bent over and gave him a farewell hug, "Good luck, Ted. And, don't forget about us."

Weak—but not down-for-the count—his counts were actually pretty good, Ted was ready to continue to fight. He held his arm out for Brenda to steady him, as he stepped over the threshold and into his home. There were no banners of success strung across the door, no balloons bobbing with "Congratulations," and no bands playing *We Will, We Will, Rock You.* There were only signs of the hard work ahead. His "bag of goodies" carried pills, doctors' instructions, and a long list of do's and don'ts. He set them on the dining room table. At the top of his "do list" was to sit in his La-Z-Boy recliner. Like his dog Jesse, Teddy sniffed around the living room for his favorite cushion and surrendered to the soft, black leather. His waif of a butt had found its way home and he reached for the remote.

Ted may have been home, but where was that? Loudon, New Hampshire. His family was there, but what about his sense of identity? He hadn't worked in months. Employee friends kept in touch, but it wasn't the same. He had missed so much while he was absent. What would happen if he couldn't go back to work? These were obstacles he took seriously. Ativan helped him sleep nights when anxiety about his future kept him wide awake. And, he didn't want to ask for help—it was not his nature.

The ability to help someone is a gift especially when the help is not asked for. I'm sure Teddy didn't want to ask for help, in the same way that a few of his dairy farmers didn't want to. When Ted was a dairy inspector he encountered unsavory, born-and-bred New Englanders, who were nastier than "suckin' hind tits." They didn't want any young bumpkin, know-it-all, from the government messing with their farms. Though he was an "outsider" to them, Ted had an insider's working knowledge that came in handy. It created conflict that sometimes couldn't be avoided. One old bastard came at him with a hammer. Teddy sloughed it off saying, "The poor guy has issues. It wasn't right to make matters worse."

For months Teddy warned one of the farmers on his route that he was going to have to shut him down.

"Sir, I can't keep letting you get by without a hand sink in your milk room."

"Boy, I have more important things to worry about."

"But, I can't keep lookin' the other way. It's important to have a hand sink for sanitary reasons."

"For reasons I ain't gonna share with you, I haven't been able to get to it. You think I have time to run around fixin' up the milk room when I got other chores to do?"

"I know it must be tough, but I am gonna have to close you down if you don't get a sink in here."

Uncomfortable with conflict, Teddy devised a solution. He took a trip to a local dump and scouted around until he found an old bathroom sink. Then, he went to the hardware store and bought some copper pipe. He went back to his farm and installed the wash sink himself. Ted didn't shut him down.

At home, Ted continued to suffer from residual fatigue, dizziness, nausea, sporadic fevers, and a lack of balance. He fell while he was out at the clothesline. Teddy bounced his body off the walls, and redirected himself to the bathroom in the middle of the night. The darkness presented a new set of challenges, and a physical therapist had to help him with "orientation exercises." Standing on one foot, Teddy practiced balancing in his living room. When he felt up to it, he ventured outside. Mom arrived on one visit only to find Ted in his garden hoeing. He wasn't supposed to be playing in the dirt. The sight took her by surprise.

"Ted, what are you doing?"

Pants drooping in the afternoon sun, he stood gripping the wooden pole with both hands. He replied, "The hoe helps me with my balance." But, that wasn't Mom's point.

"When you were little, it was a struggle to get you to hoe a few rows in the strawberry patch and now you're out here in your condition. Weren't you instructed to stay away from things that could carry germs?"

At eleven years old, I envied the floppy, red flannel hat that Teddy wore into the garden to weed. Plus, he didn't have to wear a shirt. Weeding the strawberry plants early in the day meant we might get to go to the island. But now, we had our jobs to do. I found my two long rows of bushy, leaf-covered plants, with shoots like miniature squids that reached from one cluster to the next. I spotted one large, shiny red berry drooping toward the ground. In my dungaree shorts, bare feet, and red and black paisley sleeveless shirt, I plunked myself down at the beginning of the first row. White flowers peeking between green leaves made an arch across the dirt. I tried not to sit on them. Teddy knelt down a few rows to my right and started lightly pelting me with tiny dirt bombs. These were not like the huge dirt bomb that he launched at our much younger sister Dolly. That dirt bomb filled up one of her eyes and made her look like a pirate without a patch. (Teddy felt real bad about that one.) I hunched my shoulders, ducked my head, and tried to ignore him. Bored, he gave up. I brushed the dirt clumps out of my hair and dug my fingers into the yielding, brown earth. I pulled up a good clump of weeds.

Teddy searched for ways to make it through each day. He pulled one pant leg on at a time. There was no need to comb his hair. He didn't have any. His familiar baseball cap went with him on his walks. Mom, Dad, and I went with him when we could.

Mom was there to help Ted when he needed an infusion at Dartmouth. She stayed over the night before so that Brenda could drop them off at the hospital. Brenda needed to go to work. She had taken considerable time away from her job already. Dr. Bates told Ted he needed to double his amount of fluid intake and ordered a four-hour hydration infusion. Hydration infusion—this was something new. In addition to this, he could have had a blood transfusion but Ted wanted to give his own red blood cells a chance to rejuvenate. Mom called Dad to ask him to pick them up at 2:00 PM and I got word that Dad was going to make the two-hour drive alone.

Dad was working his Tuesday morning schedule at the East Kingston Town Hall. To keep himself active, as if he wasn't active enough, he helped out as the Selectmen's assistant. He'd been at it for years. I was working, too, that day, and had to do an errand in East Kingston. I went to his office. Dad's "office girls" knew that he was worried and they were hesitant to make eye contact with me. With brows more furrowed than usual and eyes downcast, Dad got up from his desk and strode over to the counter.

"What are you doing here?"

"Did you want me to drive you up to Dartmouth?"

Drumming the counter with his fingers, he paused, "I can do it."

"I know, Dad, but would you like me to go along?" Help—when to give it, when to offer it, when to ask for it, and when to accept it—sometimes it's tough to call. I knew that Dad could make the drive, but after all he was seventy-eight-years old. His son was, as they say in the American Cancer Society, "living with cancer."

"I'm thinking maybe I should go with you."

"Maybe so." Dad was fine with me driving but still asked, "Aren't you working today?"

"Yes, but I think I'll call my boss and let her know I think it's important that I drive you up to Dartmouth."

"Whatever you think is best."

"That's what I'm going to do."

"Okay, I'll get out a little early today. Do you want to have lunch with me before we go?"

"Sure. I'll meet you back at the house."

I sat in my car for a few minutes weighing the situation—torn between my responsibility to work and my responsibility to family. Family won. There were times when work had won out and I had lived to regret it. So, maybe I didn't absolutely, positively have to drive Dad to Dartmouth. Maybe Dad and Mom and Ted could have done all right without me. Maybe, I needed to do this for me. I called my boss on my cell phone. "Hi, I really feel I need to drive my dad to pick up Ted this afternoon at Dartmouth."

"That's fine, Lucinda. Do whatever you need to do." It helped that she understood.

Teddy was just about finished by the time we got to the outpatient treatment center. A nurse was giving him last minute instructions. He was putting bottles filled with pills into his bag. As I looked over the room with white curtains drawn, nurses going from patient to patient, and Ted's empty, white, sheet-covered chair—I thought I was in a foreign country. I was a foreigner; and flying monkeys might as well be carrying little dogs, for as much as what I saw made sense to me. Wizard, I wish Teddy could click his heels three times and wake up from this terrible dream.

"Are you ready Ted?"

"Yeah. Did you have any trouble parking?"

"No. I actually lucked out. When I was driving around the corner of the parking lot, this lady was taking off. I got a good space right in front of the hospital."

"That's good."

It was good because every step Teddy took was calculated. It was painful to watch. In their late seventies Mom and Dad should have been the "slow walkers," but they could have raced to the lobby and back a couple times over before Ted could reach the front doors. (Remembering *The Hobbit...he would have been ashes before he took his second step.*) And, when it came time to getting him in the car, it was as if I was helping one of my ninety-year old residents on an outing from the retirement home. I guarded the top of my silver Chrysler Sebring, making sure he didn't bang his head. Patiently, I waited for him to lift up his leg with both hands under his thigh and place his foot on the mat. Dad and Mom sat in the back so he wouldn't get car sick. We let him sleep all the way home.

Fortunately, most of his dizziness subsided—which allowed him to take a walk outside with us before we had to get back to East Kingston. Ted measured the distance from his driveway to the top of the hill and back—another way to keep track of his progress. On good days, he could go a little farther and watch the new development going up. On not-so-good days he didn't make it out of the house.

I never even knew there was a new development. The four of us meandered up the road, on-guard in case Teddy lost his balance. We were worried he would fall at any moment. We took turns spotting.

At the top of the hill, I thought Teddy had probably gone far enough, but he wasn't changing direction. "Do you want to keep going?"

"Yeah, just a bit farther. I'll show you the new development."

"You sure?"

"Yup."

We continued to the stop sign and then across to the unpaved road. One over-sized home with two floors was sided up to the bow windows, and a "For Sale" sign was posted in the yard. Construction workers had left for the day, but heavy trucks were parked along the side of the street.

"How long has this been goin' on? I didn't even know there was a road this far up." I had never gone beyond his driveway.

"It's been under construction for awhile now."

"It seems like you've been living here forever. How long has it been?"

"Let's see, we moved here in 1985. You and Pat stayed at that campground with Matt and Mandy so Pat could help me with the framing. That was a big help."

"Well, you helped us with our house."

A motley crew—strong, but without professional carpentry experience—assembled on our property the day we unloaded the pine purlins, long, continuous beams that run from one end of the log supported roof to the other. It took ten men, two on each side, to carry nine massive beams out of the long-body truck and place them in the front yard. Again, I was on camera duty. It was Memorial Day 1978. Dad Clark, Pat's dad, brother-in-law Dave, and even John Keeley, the one who crashed heads with Teddy in the basketball game, agreed to help us with this hernia-producing work. Dave grimaced on one side of the beam while John leaned over smiling. Pat and his dad heaved it up to shoulder height, as Teddy and Jimmy led the beam off the truck. I worried but no one got hurt.

"Yeah. That was back when I was single."

"It was a lot of work."

"But, we had fun doin' it."

"I know—we have beer can drainage around the foundation to prove it."

"You know it's Kevin's birthday today."

"I'm sorry. I forgot all about that. How old is he?"

"Fifteen. Imagine that. And Corey graduates from high school this Saturday," Ted's voice cracked as he spoke about his son's graduation.

We turned at the "For Sale" sign and headed back down the hill. Silently, Mom, Dad, and I hoped that Ted would be able to make it to the big graduation party on June 28, 2003. It was a combined celebration for Jim's son Tyler and Ted's son Corey.

Always remember, when your heart needs lifting—think of happy thoughts—a pipe, garden at twilight, June under the stars, and a son's graduation. With a new walking stick, instead of a sword, Ted attended Corey's graduation. He was dizzy and thin, but he was smiling when Corey walked down the aisle and received his diploma. Ted may have partied a little too hard, because he paid for it the next day.

He called Mom, "Thanks for comin' to Corey's graduation."

"We are very proud of him. Glad we could go. How are you doin' today?"

"So. So. I've got some cold symptoms and I'm feelin' a little sick."

During the week, he came down with a cold and continued to be dizzy but he did begin to eat better. He managed to drive Kevin to play rehearsal in Plaistow and go for a two-mile walk to Becky's house. By Saturday, he was well enough to participate in Tyler's and Corey's graduation party.

Jim's wife sent the party invitation a month before. It was imprinted with a collage of photos. One photo was of Jim with his baby boy. Another was of Ted with his baby boy. The handsome, smiling, professional graduation pictures of Corey and Tyler graced the left margin of the invitation. In the upper right corner was an oval-shaped snapshot of Ted with his hands in his pockets and Corey, peeking over his left shoulder, strapped to his back. Jim, with Tyler on his back, was resting his arm on a brown, wooden sign in between them. It read: Mt. Kearsarge, Elev. 2937 ft., Trail To Summit, 5 miles.

It was a beautifully done invitation; one that Jim's wife must have put a lot of thought into. It impressed me at the time but it impresses me even more now, as I read the inscription at the top, "Within every celebrated ending, a new opportunity beckons." And, at the bottom, "Within every ending there lies a new beginning that beckons us to reach out and explore." Tyler and Corey were ending their high school years, and about to explore a world outside the boundaries of their parents. Teddy was ending another round of cancer treatment and about to find out about what new beginning was in store for him. It was time to celebrate endings and embrace new opportunities.

In the spirit of Clark family tradition, nothing is done in small quantities. Jimmy rented a tent and prepared for the onslaught of guests, carrying banquet-sized tables and fifty folding chairs onto the front lawn. Friends and family arrived on foot, riding bikes, and in cars and vans. Bumper kissed bumper in their driveway. Coolers of food and drink lined the edges of the tent. Large grills snapped from hamburger grease. Aunts and uncles mingled with nieces and nephews. "I haven't seen you in a while," hung in the air until someone caught it and ran with it. No one was more happy to be there than Teddy.

Wearing a green baseball cap and a blue collared short-sleeve shirt, he leaned on his walking stick and climbed up the small hill to the meeting ground. Although his pale, aged skin and sunken, facial features resembled our great grandpa Simeon, Ted's smile was as contagious as ever. He was up to his usual tricks—making fun of Muffy's famous fudge, and the way Jimmy ran back and forth from the house. Ted was content to be alive. Mom and Dad couldn't be happier that we were all there, all seven of their children. Dad needed a picture. He approached me first.

"I want to get a picture of the seven of you with Mom and me."

"But, Dad, I have to leave with Mandy," I had already stayed longer than I planned and I was getting fidgety, "We have to go to her friend's wedding and it's in Concord."

"It'll only take a minute."

"Dad, it'll take twenty minutes just to get everyone together."

My eyes swam across a sea of related faces and surfaced on my siblings. They were bobbing here and there. They were brightly colored species that shimmered amongst the ordinary school of fish. Short Muffy, affectionately nicknamed "hostess with the mostess," was in a hot debate with an aunt and uncle under the far end of the tent. Her flailing arm almost knocked the drink out of a cousin's passing hand. Party-planning Becky, who hosted the annual Yankee swap, was listening to a conversation, outside the tent between another cousin and his wife. Becky was probably planning Labor Day weekend. By Jimmy's pool, decisive Debbie, who was always the one to make a decision and stick to it, was gesturing to her daughter to come speak with her aunt. Debbie was deciding how she could meet her aunt's grandson. Adorable Dolly, the "baby of the family", was laughing at a family story while Teddy looked on. They were in the middle of the tent. Energetic Jim, who was always up early and raring to go, was "as frantic as a rooster in a hen house" trying to make sure there was enough food. He kept asking, "Are you getting enough to eat?" I figured it would be hopeless to get them to stop what they were doing. "It'll take too long. Just take the picture without me."

"Oh, come on. It won't take that long." The look that flashed across Dad's face made me think twice. I excused myself and plowed through the tent, tapping Dolly on the elbow and looking at Ted, "Dad wants a picture of all of us. I don't have much time, so go over by the pool." They could see I was in a hurry, "Gee, Dolly, I guess she means business." They headed for the pool while I recruited Becky to get Muffy—who would be the most difficult to stop from talking. Debbie was already near the pool. As soon as we gathered, Dad told us what to do.

"Line up in front of the pool. Mom and I will kneel in front." We started to get in a line but it wasn't the way Dad wanted, "Line up in birth order." In the commotion to get this done quickly, Debbie was squeezing in between Jimmy and me. She should have been between Becky and Muffy. Ted piped up, "That's okay... I have a new birthday anyway." We laughed, thinking that was pretty clever of him. Dad let it go. The picture was taken—Becky, Muffy, Teddy, Cindy, Debbie, Jimmy, and Dolly—the first and last time a family photo was taken that way.

Soon after that party in June, Ted and I went on our respective vacations. The four thousand kilometers southwest of Hawaii it took Pat and me to fly to Tahiti on July 2, 2003 was vast. It was comparable to the travel Ted made, from his diagnosis on August 7, 2002 to Bar Harbor, Maine on that same Fourth of July weekend. Both were momentous occasions that brought Ted and me to remote locations. It took work and a kind of commitment to the unknown to arrive at these destinations. In the months leading up to our trip, I kept wondering if Pat and I would have to cancel our plans. We took out travel insurance just in case. Ted wondered if he would make it to the next month. (My mom and dad made sure that Ted's life insurance bill was paid.) Thirty years of marriage was something to celebrate. Pat and I worked hard at reaching thirty years together, just as Ted worked hard in his fight for his life.

Though the shores of Bora Bora and the shores of Bar Harbor, Maine are oceans apart, Teddy was in my heart and with me in spirit. I never stopped thinking about him. The darker, deeper blues and lighter hues of Maine's salty, numbing water captivated Ted in the same way the aqua blue and pastel greens of Bora Bora's less salty, warm water fascinated me. The rich layers of ocean colors reflected different composition—equally beautiful.

Over the years, Ted and I went our separate ways. (Brenda and I went our separate ways as well.) He went off to college and then, came back. He went off to Colorado and then, came back. He went off to the hospital and then, came back. In a way, I never left home. Eventually,

Ted always came crashing in. I counted on that but I never took it for granted.

To the east Ted was preparing to go for a late afternoon walk. With effort, because of the numbness in his fingers, he laced his sneakers. He sat on the steps of his Bar Harbor retreat and listened to his boys still inside.

"Kevin, you're so lazy. Why don't you get out and do somethin'?" Corey was determined to get Kevin out of the house.

"What business is it of yours? So what if I'm not like you. I like video games rather than runnin' around and bikin'." Kevin had his usual come-back.

"It seems like you're wastin' your life sittin' around doin' nothin'." Corey wasn't giving up.

"It may seem like nothin' to you, but I like it." Kevin made his point.

Corey gave up on talking at him and came at him—he wrapped him in a bear hug and wrestled him to the floor. Teddy ignored the loud crash as he watched Brenda take off for an ocean-side run. He called after her, "You better get your run in or we'll all suffer." Ted swayed a bit as he stood and started down the road to the country store. Perhaps he could join her in a run by next year. At any rate, there was incentive to get to the end of the day—lobster was on the horizon.

The last rays of the golden summer sun signaled time to gather the lobster paraphernalia—picks, crackers, and bibs. Click, click, click, lobsters scratched against the cooler. A lobster feast was something Ted could really sink his teeth into. (He had corrective surgery done on his teeth the year before.) He held a squiggling lobster up to Corey's face and watched him jump back.

"You want to put this big, ugly guy in the water?"

"No, Dad, you're havin' way too much fun. I'll let you do it."

With fake squealing "Eeeek, eeek, eeek," Ted dropped the lobster into the boiling pot and reached for the next one. In twenty minutes, everyone grabbed a seat and crowded around the table.

Corey and Kevin cracked the tough shells with their bare hands and flung the sharp body parts into a big bowl in the middle of the table. Green, rubbery entrails slopped on top of a mounting pile of red-orange carcasses. Lobster juice soaked newspaper covering the tablecloth. Manners were minimal as talking, laughing, and story-telling interrupted the devouring of lobster after lobster.

"'Member when Kevin..., 'member when Corey..., 'member when Mom...., 'member when Dad....."

A trickle of butter ran down Ted's chin, as he elbowed Kevin, "Hey, look at that big bird." He motioned toward the window and Kevin looked up from his plate. Teddy snatched a prime piece of lobster tail and popped it into his mouth. Kevin knew he had been taken, "Dad...I was saving that one for last."

To the west I was pulling into the dock. I knew I wasn't in Kingston anymore. The sight of over-water bungalows planted on stilts above tranquil turquoise water took my breath away. I never thought I would get this far—a tear trickled down my cheek. Pat, ever familiar with my erratic emotion, could see it coming as a slight breeze brushed it away. The pointed, thatched roofs and sleeping accommodations looked like triangular shaped umbrellas, protecting square, light brown boxes with round wooden legs. They did not resemble anything in Bar Harbor. I searched for ours—at the far end of a long, wooden pier. A land pyramid of dark green vegetation and rocky formations loomed in the background—a Motu. A few friendly, white clouds drifted in the brilliant, blue sky and the air smelled fresh and clean.

July fourth was like any other day in Bora Bora. As the captain motioned us to depart the boat, deliciously warm wind whipped across my face and welcomed me to the island. As fire crackers rocketed over the shores of Bar Harbor, I wrapped my senses around this scene and wondered to myself, "What would Teddy think if he could see me now?"

Ted gained ten to twelve pounds and his blood counts continued to rise. By the beginning of August, he was well enough to go kayaking with Dad.

"Where do you want to go?" Dad asked.

"I don't care. Where did you have in mind?" Ted asked.

"We could go along the Pow Wow or we could go out on Kingston Lake," Dad answered.

"I guess it shouldn't be very busy on a Monday morning. Let's go to Kingston. I haven't been there in years," Ted replied.

Ted took charge and drove his Explorer with two kayaks strapped to the roof. He backed out of the driveway and they chatted briefly on the way to Kingston.

"I wonder how Skippy's doin'," Teddy thought out loud.

Skippy kept up a steady vigil, calling and visiting regularly, with him from the day he was diagnosed. They were close. As children,

Skippy lived just a short walk away. Running, it took less than eight minutes. They played football together. They rode motorcycles together. Skip's father owned the island where they water-skied, showing off in front of Kingston State Park. I hated "to spot" for Skippy and Teddy.

I gripped the slippery, white, fiberglass of the Boston Whaler—traveling thirty-five mph. Skippy held the steering wheel tight and dodged an oncoming motorboat pulling another water-skier. He swerved toward Kingston State Park. We hit a washboard of waves and a "double-up," that sent me ricocheting off my seat. I jammed my hand between my knee and the wave-soaked boat cushion. Recovering from that set of waves, I braced for the next one. I leaned to the right and then to the left as Skippy hit the throttle even harder. I concentrated on Teddy through the arcs of water, an arc to the right and then to the left, as he crossed both wakes at full speed. Biceps bulging, he forced the rope up over his head, arched his back and administered a boat-moving yank.

As he steered his ski in the opposite direction he buckled at the waist and lost control ending up in a full-face plant. I felt the lurch in the boat as Teddy let go of the rope and disappeared under the water. His ski rocketed off him and landed far to his right.

"He's down," I yelled to Skippy over the motor.

Skippy cut the engine and started to redirect the boat. As he pulled closer to Teddy's submerged body, I leaned over the side of the boat, "Are you goin' again?"

Teddy whipped his wet hair out of his eyes and squirted water out of his mouth. He reached for the wooden handle, at the end of the rope, as it drifted toward him.

"Yeah. Take me back to the island."

I watched as he ducked his head under the water and wrestled to get his ski back on. We had to circle back one more time to bring the handle close enough for him to grab. He held it tight with both hands and lined the tip of his ski up with the back of the boat.

As loud as he could, he yelled to Skippy, "Hit it!"

It struck Skip hard when Ted was diagnosed with cancer.

"I know Skippy has been workin' hard on redoin' the garage," Dad said to Ted as they drove near the building.

"Yeah. He told me about that the last time he came up to visit. I haven't seen it yet, though." Ted was interested in the renovation.

Dad and Ted pulled in at the family-owned, Clark's—pronounced 'Clahk's by a senior aunt—garage. The carport, framed in brick and arched with solid wood panels painted white, looked the same as it did in the early 1900s, a fixture along The Plains. They peeked in the front office but everyone had gone to lunch. Teddy got back in his Explorer and drove by the oil tank and through the narrow alley. He ignored the "Do Not Trespass" sign dragging from a chain. He continued on down the dirt road that led to the lake. I doubt he was thinking about how he taught me to drive a Honda 350 motorcycle along that very road.

"CC—you wanna' drive it?" Teddy asked.

It hadn't occurred to me, watching him spin around the back road, that he would want me to drive his manly-man's bike. I was comfortable sitting on the back. The deep, pumpkin-colored tank with a standard black and white Honda logo had barely a scratch. I'm not sure why he did. His question caught me off guard but I didn't wait for him to change his mind.

"What do I do?"

His instructions were about as explicit as teaching me how to grab the farm rope tow.

"Hold the bike steady." He showed me first by example, straddling the bike and holding the handle bars with both hands. "Let out the clutch, while you give it some gas." He showed me the controls. "When you feel it start to grab, let yourself go and give it more gas." He took off down the road, spun around in the pull-off, and came back. He hit the brakes before hitting my feet. He showed me how to use the brakes, then sliding off the bike gestured for me to get on. He waited for me to mount it before he let go.

I wasn't expecting it to be so heavy! As I held the handlebars I felt the weight of this machine press against my left leg. It was starting to fall. I braced myself against it and yanked it back upright. That made my hands shake, but Teddy didn't notice.

"Just hold it tight," he said.

"Sure, Ted, why didn't you tell me this thing weighs a ton?" I asked disgusted.

"Don't be a coward, you can do it." He urged me on.

I gripped the handlebars firmer and steadied the bike. Girlishly, I let out the clutch and gave it the gas; naturally it did a hiccup and came to a halt. Grinning, Teddy showed me how to do it again. This time, I let the clutch out slowly and allowed the engine to engage. I felt the wheels move under me, saw the trees starting to pass by me, heard the roar of the engine, and smelled the exhaust. I let out a little scream. You might say, "I felt the earth move under my feet, I felt the sky tumbling down…"

Teddy took all the sharp turns on the way to the lake, observing the antique bottle-infested valley on the right and a new house in the clearing. The woods on either side were still pretty thick, but "Do Not Trespass" didn't stop stray campers from Kingston State Park from entering the private property. Beer bottles and Funny Bone wrappers were strewn along the ground. He drove down the last hill filled with ruts and parked next to the lone aging birch.

Dad and Ted took turns helping each other lift the kayaks off the roof and carried them to the lake. There were only a few canoes and a few motorboats drifting around the edges. There wasn't a cloud in the sky. One water-skier could be seen in the distance on the other side of the lake by Camp Lincoln. Dad held Ted's kayak against the dock as it began to tip.

"I'll steady it for you." Dad reached over to help.

"I got it." Ted didn't need it.

The effects of Ted's year of cancer treatment and Dad's advanced age made them an even match. As they paddled away from shore Ted pulled ahead. He methodically dipped his paddle into the water on one side of the boat, and then the other. He wasn't trying to come in first in the Lamprey River canoe race. Dad caught up, staying just out of paddle touching distance, as they headed to the island, kayaks skimming the water.

They paddled across the lake in front of Kingston State Park, and then glided along the fringe of Clark's Island. Branches dropped twigs on their heads. Trees, shrubs, and bushes, covered the large land mass from east to west, and north to south. The dense growth made it difficult to walk across the island, except where there were paths. It was the only island on the lake. It was recognizable from various shore lines. Ted made his way around the tip of the island that would bring him to the ski cove. Dad followed. He drew close enough to gaze up the steep incline and see the green, shingled porch with brown and white trim. The two story cottage with intricate details and a narrow, wooden staircase was the only building on the entire acreage. The old cottage still guarded the point.

How many nights had Skippy and he slept in the upper, front bedroom facing the lake? How many times had he slid down the hill of pine needles, with ski jacket and ski in his hands? How many white, metal buckets of water had he carried up the hill to flush the out-house toilet? How many cousins, siblings, aunts, and uncles, had done these very same things? It was too many to count, but it did matter. Ted was no island.

Mom called to let everyone know, "Ted has shingles." The first thing I thought of was that older people typically get it. That is, unless one happens to be HIV infected, immunosuppressed, or be a patient receiving cancer treatments. Red blisters break out under the skin that causes a burning or tingling sensation. The condition can be relatively painful. In Ted's case it was a pain in the butt. Like everything else, he took it in stride. The neurologist confirmed that he had inner-ear damage and neuropathy in his feet.

On the plus side, therapy was helping his balance and his blood work continued to show improvement. In between kayaking and taking Kevin to play practices Ted took his medication. On August 20th, Ted had yet another CT scan. He waited eight days for his appointment at Dartmouth Hitchcock to hear the results in person. "Ted, we are cautiously optimistic. We believe you are in remission." This news came three days before Becky's Labor Day Weekend party. There would be more to celebrate than the fifteen August and September birthdays of various family members.

We were all cautiously optimistic. Ted had received good news but how good was it? It was real and it was good, but it wasn't real good. Cautiously, Becky decided to make a sign recognizing Ted's achievement. In bold letters it read, "TED, YOU MADE IT, MIRACLES HAPPEN." She stuck it in the ground near the top of the steps, leading to her front door. She attached balloons—one white, one blue, and one pink on the left side; one red and one yellow on the right. They floated toward the west. Bright, red geraniums accented the lower left corner of the sign. I watched Ted walk up the stairs. He stopped in front of it. I could see his eyes begin to tear and his bottom lip begin to quiver. A Bar Harbor gust of wind could have knocked him over. I was standing on the front steps and stayed grounded until he came closer.

"How was your trip to Bar Harbor?"

"It was great."

"How was your trip to Bora Bora?"

"It was great."

King of the Forest

For a brief time in the fall of 2003, Ted held onto the belief that his cancer was in remission. He had the chance to live like he was dying; and he did what he could do. Once again, he went bike riding.

Ted, Brenda, Pat, and I had ridden our bikes from East Kingston to Hampton Beach; Jimmy and Teddy had ridden together in Canada, in Maine, and all over New Hampshire; Brenda and Ted had ridden all over Loudon. Brenda and I had ridden around Lake Fairlee, but this was different. When I had my last supper with my dancing buddy Abigail, I knew it could be the last time. In the same way, I knew this could be my last bike ride with Teddy. I took this day for what it was—today for Ted, tomorrow for me. I tried to take note of every detail even though I'm not a person who likes to focus on details. An angel's in these details. When I was in the middle of hard labor, I gripped the bed rails and forced myself to remember what it felt like just in case I thought about getting pregnant again. When I was on this bike ride, I savored every sensation so that I could remember what it felt like just in case it didn't happen again. I needed this memory to play over, and over, and over again. When Ted and Brenda drove into Dad's driveway, with their bikes strapped to the roof, Jim and I were ready.

"Don't you look snappy," I couldn't help but give Jimmy the business about his choice of clothing, "You'd think you were a professional racer or something. Where's your pack of Camels?" I knew it was a camel pack but was busting his balls. He was wearing a tight blue biker's shirt with fluorescent pink designs. Even his daughters would have to admit he was looking pretty hot.

Jim tilted his sunglasses and smiled, "Don't you ever wear something besides that old sweatshirt?"

I countered, "Hey, this is my good luck Georgia Tech sweatshirt. Don't be messin' with that."

Ted, in his casual, tan, long sleeve shirt, leaned on his handle bars and squinted toward Jim, "Gee, Jim, I forgot to bring my sunglasses."

Light shone through the maples by the rock wall and made a stripe across the front of Brenda's yellow fluorescent jacket, "Let's go before it gets too late." She clipped her shoes into the brackets and pointed her bike toward the road, "We're going to Newton, right?" She was off before I had a chance to start a conversation with her.

To fill in the gaps (Teddy didn't like "gaposis," the expression he used for the gaps in between his woodworking projects) Ted took a bush whacker and bush-hogged the field in front of Dad's barn. The fresh air of the fall day revived some of his strength and made him look much better. At night he watched his son, Kevin, perform in the *Mikado*. Though acting was far removed from what Ted would ever have done, he was proud of his son. Kevin was a standout. The only acting Ted had done was in "Cousin Capers." With a pillowcase draped over his head and two eyes, a nose, and mouth drawn on his stomach, he stepped onto the stage in the upstairs of the Pilgrim Church. The occasion was Mom's seventieth birthday. Everyone was asked to make a fool of themselves, and he was no exception. Like everyone else that participated in this celebration, he was a good sport. His belly button, painted with red lipstick, sucked in and out to whistling, along with three other male cousins. To this day, the thought of it makes me laugh!

The four of us agreed to ride to Newton, swing through parts of Kingston then head back to East Kingston. No one was counting but it would be a slow ten miles or so. Teddy and I, consciously or unconsciously, held back as Jimmy took off. He popped a wheelie over the knoll on the way out of the upper driveway, stood up pedaling a few feet to the lower driveway and jammed on his brakes—spinning around sideways and then to a stop. He looked back at us chuckling at his own expense, "I had to try out my new brakes."

Teddy and I swerved our tires toward the rock wall, then back toward the road and tried to ignore him, "Yeah right."

We rode in tandem, Brenda and Jim in the front and Ted and I in the back. We pedaled down Willow Road and out to Route 107. Passing the old Turkey Farm, I called out to Ted, "Remember when Rick Santos came and stayed with you?" Rick, from the Fresh Air Program, stayed with us one summer.

"I remember he didn't like strawberries. Can you believe that?" Even Ted thought that was strange.

"I know, but at least he didn't come at you with a carving knife like Sadie Billingham did," I hollered over to him.

Teddy was always jumping out from behind a door to scare the bejesus out of me. I was used to it. It was a habit that I picked up from him and passed on to Jimmy. Any one of us could be guilty of it. Sadie Billingham, an eleven-year-old girl from Dorchester, MA, came to live with us for two weeks one summer. She told me about the rats that crawled out from the holes in their tenement building at 1:00 in the morning, about how she pulled the fire alarm and watched the fire trucks come, and about her life in the city with her twelve brothers and sisters. They didn't go around spooking each other just for the fun of it.

Sadie, in a world of her own, hummed to herself as she came step by step down the stairs in our front hallway. I slid behind the living room door and waited. She was smiling as she hit the red, worn rug. I shouted, "Booo!!" Well, Sadie's skinny black arms and black legs started shaking so bad, I thought they were going to detach from her body. She screamed so loud it pierced my eardrums. It took me fifteen minutes to calm her down. I wasn't about to do that again. But, Teddy did.

Sadie and I never told Teddy about the spooking incident. A few days later, Sadie and I were setting the table for supper. Teddy, chuckling to himself, crawled on the floor behind the kitchen counter, unnoticed by Sadie and me. As she was heading for the table with a white dinner plate, he popped up in front of her. When he did, Sadie's eyes crazed over, and shot flecks of red and white light in Teddy's face. The plate fell, smashing into bits and pieces. Her shrill, neighbor-reaching shriek was so loud it brought Mom running from the dining room. Teddy jumped back. He knocked over a chair and landed on the floor. Instinctively, Sadie grabbed a long, sharp knife from the edge of the sink and held it high above him. She threatened to stab him. Mom closed in on Sadie to try to reason with her, "Sadie, please stop! Sadie, please stop!"

Sadie unclasped her child-strong fist and let the knife drop. On the way to the floor, it glanced off a silver drawer pull and nicked Teddy's bent knee. It twirled one last time before its tip ended with a metallic thud. Teddy and I had never seen a knife held in anger, but perhaps Sadie had.

We rounded the corner after Jewett's General store and started toward Newton. I pedaled close enough to Ted to try to carry on with conversation.

"When do you think you'll be able to go back to work?" My question was drowned by a passing maroon Dodge caravan.

"What?" Ted didn't hear me the first time.

"When are you planning to go back to work?" I asked him again.

"The first of October." He sounded matter-of-fact.

Only the round, fluorescent light over the kitchen table was on when Teddy drove into the gravelly driveway. He scuffed his boots on the rug and opened the door. Closing the kitchen door, the first thing he did was turn to the left and look at the blackboard. "We've gone to bed. There's left-over roast beef and mashed potatoes in the frig. Leave some for the rest of us for lunch tomorrow. John called."

Teddy pulled the bench away from the table, sat down, and began to conjure a plan. Rubbing his hands together, like the Wicked Witch of the East, he looked into his crystal ball. He could see Jimmy driving alone up Scotland Road. With the toe end of his left boot, Teddy tugged at the back of his right heel. He kicked off his crusty work boot. It hit the wood box, landing on its side. He did the same with his opposite foot—his long, dingy-white sock left a trail of hay from the bench to the wood box. He took both hands and ripped away his grimy-white t-shirt, finishing off the large tear that had already started beneath his collar bone. He wrapped it into a ball and, as if shooting a basketball, aimed for the wastebasket. It hit the backboard, the end of the counter, and landed in the trash. He was thinking about Jimmy coming home.

Like a burglar, doing his burgling, Teddy shut off the one remaining light. He looked out the window. It was dark next door. He watched until he saw two bright lights shining on the cement well cover. As Jimmy slammed the car door, Teddy tiptoed into the bathroom and slipped past the sink. He climbed on top of the toilet seat behind the door and crouched over, as if a large cat getting ready to pounce. He knew Jimmy would have to pee when he came in.

Aware that everyone had gone to bed, Jimmy quietly crossed the kitchen floor and headed straight for the bathroom. In the dark, he bumped into the door frame and fumbled for the light switch. Just as light illuminated the mirror above the sink, Teddy jumped off the toilet seat, shouting "Boo!" Jimmy was an attacked cat. He let out a prey's fierce scream—ready to scratch Teddy's eyes out. The cat-like screech should have woken our neighbor. Jimmy contracted his paws and pounded, out of control, on Teddy's bare chest. He knocked the mirror off the wall and it made a terrible crash. Teddy just stood there. After a flurry of punches and the shock starting to wear off, Jimmy came to his senses and realized he was staring face to face with his brother. Jimmy hauled off one last hit for good measure before they both went into hysterics, tears rolling down their cheeks.

Instead of going back to work, Ted went back to the doctors. On September 30th he was at Dartmouth Hospital having a CT scan and bone marrow biopsies from both hips. He learned the next day that his bone marrow was fine, but there was a small spot that showed up on the CT scan. This would require a PET scan.

Pat's mom and dad were anxious for Ted to get better. When I glided down their driveway with Ted nearly bumping into my back tire, they were not expecting us.

"Well, this is a surprise." Dad Woodbury, with his size fifteen shoes, leaving man-prints in the grass, strode over to Ted, "Ted, how are you?"

"Great. It's good to see you." Ted smiled up at him.

"It sure is great to see you, too. Where are you guys goin'?" Dad Woodbuy aked.

"Just around the old neighborhood. We might go down New Boston Road next."

"You might not recognize some of the new development."

"It's goin' on everywhere."

Jimmy slid down the hill, straddled his bike, and broke into the conversation, he asked, "How's Suzie doin'?" (Jimmy was in the same class as Suzie, Pat's sister.)

"She's doin' good, workin' hard, you know the story," Dad Woodbury said.

"I sure do. Is Eric still doin' a lot of ridin'?" Jimmy knew that Suzie's husband Eric was an avid road-bike rider.

"Oh yeah, he's signed up for some big race comin' up," Dad Woodbury answered.

As the men continued to talk, Brenda and I chatted with Mom Woodbury. Brenda wanted to know the latest on Pat's brother, "What's Tim up to?" she asked.

"The usual, he's workin' lots of hours and tryin' to fit in some fishin' at Plum Island on the weekends," Mom Woodbury answered without hesitation.

"I love the ocean. Ted and I should take a ride down there some day." Brenda drifted for the moment.

"How's he doin'?" Mom Woodbury glanced toward Ted.

"He's doin' pretty good," Brenda assured.

"Would you all like somethin' to drink?" Mom Woodbury asked.

We had water bottles and didn't intend to stay long, "No thanks. We're all set. I think we've stopped long enough. Besides, we can't keep Jimmy in one place too long, he'll drive us all nuts," I said casually, glancing in his direction.

Jimmy was bouncing his front tire up and down on the tar, so I got my bike under me and I pushed up the hill. Brenda and I watched for cars as we started to pull away. Teddy pulled up the rear. Dad Woodbury called after him, "Ted, I hope you make a full recovery. We'll be thinkin' of yeah." Ted, his helmet tied securely under his chin, nodded back and gave him one thumb up.

Head down, Dad Woodbury walked toward his shed thinking, "Oh, how Ted used to muck-up on my '65' Chevy windshield." Instead of waiting for the defroster to clear away the fog, Ted rubbed his hand across the inside of the glass, leaving a big streaky mess. Pat had to take out Windex and paper towels to clean up after him, every time Pat borrowed his dad's car. It happened so often that Teddy would run his fingers across the glass, even if there wasn't any fog. Teddy knew it ticked him off. Like tapping his pencil on my desk when I was trying to study, he liked to get a reaction.

Ted called Mom on October 20th to tell her the news from Dr. Bates. The PET scan showed some uptake of isotopes in his spleen and right leg. He would need to have a biopsy of his spleen to determine if it was caused by infection, injury, or cancer. An appointment was set up.

Ted wanted to work on his bathroom but wasn't able. "Dad, you don't need to come up to help me with the bathroom. I'm not feelin' very good today."

"Do you want me to come up anyway?"

"Maybe. I'll call you around noon time."

Dad's shaky hand reached for the phone and continued to shake as he listened to his son's voice, "I'm havin' fevers and shakin' pretty bad........."

"I'll drive up and sit with you." Dad put the phone back in its place and looked to Mom.

"Hon, I'll go with you."

Ted was resting on the couch in his den when Mom and Dad arrived. Mom pulled the afghan up around his shoulders, with the same loving hands she used on me when I was sick with a migraine. Being a mother of seven children, Mom knew all about the power of healing touch. Ted had just taken some Tylenol. His eyes were closed. The obligatory ceremonies of welcoming guests were abandoned. Dad read the newspaper. Mom read her book. Teddy slept off his fever.

The leaves had started to turn—green leaves with yellowy edges flickered over our heads. The not-yet-fall air brushed across my cheeks. Mom used to send us outside to "get some fresh air." She wouldn't let us come in until our cheeks were red. As we had been taught—Teddy, Jimmy, Brenda, and I were getting our fresh air. Peaceful rays of sun followed us down New Boston Road, past the cemetery, then over the railroad tracks. We crossed over Pow Wow River and came upon the "loggin in" road, where we used to enter the woods to pick blueberries. It was on "Dad's land."

Mom dragged us into the mosquito-infested swamp abutting the Pow Wow River to search for blueberries on the muggiest day of the summer. Teddy and I dressed in long pants, long t-shirts, and our rattiest of shoes. We hung our Teddie Peanut Butter buckets from our belts and ducked under the thick bushes leading to the water's edge where tiny, dark... blue... berries were thickest. Blueberry picking etiquette says the person who finds a good bush calls to the others. I couldn't see Mom but I could hear her yell, "I've got a great one over here." I went searching for her, while Teddy stayed where he was on a hummock under a bush, munching juicy ripe berries.

"I'm goin' to catch up to Mom."

"Go ahead. I'm stayin' here."

Ted's fever subsided and he started to come out of it. He wanted to go for a walk. Mom was on one side, Dad was on the other, and Ted was in the middle. This had become a pattern. They walked slowly up the hill and checked on the progress of the new homes. It was late afternoon, just as the sun was beginning to set. Layers of rosy pinks and carnation yellows permeated the sky along the western horizon. Mom could not take her eyes off it. She watched the canvas as it changed from pleasing pastels, to lighter hues, to no color at all. She would have liked to paint it, but it was dark by the time they got back to Teddy's house.

Continuing from Newton to Kingston Ted took the lead. He pushed one leg down, pushed one leg down, and pushed one leg down, as we pedaled by the entrance to Kingston State Park. It was a good place to escape the heat on our childhood hot summer days. On July weekends, cars used to line up from our house to the gate, so dense we couldn't fit a bike in between them. Cars, mostly with Massachusetts license plates, packed with testy teenagers stalled waiting to get in. Impatient drivers honked their horns. If we couldn't go to the island, Teddy and I settled for the park.

Teddy threw his "Tony the Tiger" towel over his shoulders and tied it in a knot just under his chin. I wrapped my birthday present, a striped towel, around my waist and we ran across The Plains. I tugged at my towel trying to keep it from tripping me. By the time we reached the guard shack, I was out of breath. The brown uniformed attendant waved us through. I played hot potato on the tar on the way to the beach. In bare feet, it was a challenge to see if I could get to the first set of picnic tables, by Nason's barn, before putting my feet on the dirt. I jumped between the sun-baked tar and the rough ground. Tiny pebbles toughened my hair-covered, hobbit toes. I made funny noises all the way. Teddy was already in the water when I felt the prickly grass and then, at last, the soft sand, "Wait for me," I yelled to him. It was no use; Teddy ducked under the water and drew a deep breath. He swam under water all the way to the raft. I watched but he never came up for air. I swam after him knowing I could never hold my breath that long.

Pulling hard on one side of the ladder and then the other, water swished between my legs. I climbed up the metal steps and put my foot down on a bathing-suit clad, male-ego dominated raft. At fourteen, in a hot pink bikini, I was a prime target to get thrown in. I watched my back in order to survive the pushing, shoving, and wrestling matches that erupted around me. My wrestling days with Teddy came in handy.

Bobby grabbed me by the wrist to rocket me over the water but I whipped it down as hard and as fast as I could and yanked away. He looked surprised. I two-stepped, avoiding Jeff's oncoming arms and shoved him in the water instead. Todd snuck up behind me and gave me an aggressive two-handed push. I was going down. But, when I did, I used the "life saver" jump. Flying through the air, I spread my legs apart—left leg facing front and right leg facing back in scissor-like fashion. I made sure my arms were extended at shoulder height and braced them in a T. My head never went under. (Brenda watched from the other side of the raft.) Teddy glanced over the water and gave me a nod.

Like Bilbo Baggins, Ted could ask, *how does one survive*? On one day he was told the biopsy of his spleen did not show any signs of cancer. And, although he was having chills and fevers, he was relieved. They told him it might be an infection. On the next day he was told the call was a mistake. The team of oncologists had a conference and reversed the decision. Ted's cells were examined under a microscope. In this case, the devil was in the details. He was told, "Though we found nothing that was definitive for cancer, your history and the way you have been feeling indicates that it must be cancer. We may need to remove your spleen."

By now, Ted had learned to listen to his body and yet, he still listened to his doctors. He must have known it was his cancer returning. What would happen if he refused further treatment? He hoped they were right and he was wrong. He hoped they could solve his problem, as confusing as this was. There was no evidence-based practice for the doctors to follow. This was medical care based on speculation, gathering data, and making educated guesses. There were no hard and fast answers as to how to proceed. We were stunned, Teddy was devastated, and the doctors explored various options. The oncologists at Dartmouth Hitchcock consulted with oncology specialists at Dana Farber.

As we pedaled closer to Grammy Clark's old house, where my dad grew up, Jimmy took over the lead. Teddy was on his tail and squeezed his handbrakes as he peered into the yard. The grass was manicured and the old Colonial house was painted white with black shutters—no chipping was visible. A new picture window, free of cracks, outlined where the old kitchen once was.

Grammy Clark with her silver-white hair pulled back in a bun wrapped that baby boy in her arms and held him tight, cooing in his face. She couldn't get enough of her grandson, Teddy. She was a quintessential grandmother. She adored babies. Grammy Clark ran her index finger over his chubby knuckles and tucked her soft, wrinkled finger under his four fidgeting digits. She smiled as he curled his fingers and didn't let go. Her three baby granddaughters before him were precious too, but Teddy was the long-awaited grandson. She rocked him by the wood stove and kissed his roly-poly cheeks, singing *Rock-a-bye baby on the tree top, when the wind blows the cradle will rock...* How she must have thought of her own son Theodore John Clark. Teddy was named after him.

The first Theodore John Clark died at the age of seventeen. He was dark-haired, handsome, athletic, strong, and good-natured. I'm sure Grammy and Grampa Clark expected him to live long after them. He got a boil from the constant rubbing of his shoulder pads under his football uniform. Oddly enough, he died because this boil became infected and it could not be treated. This happened before Penicillin. (I'm wondering—will there be a miracle treatment in the future that would have cured this Theodore John Clark's cancer?)

Ted was thinking how this house has changed. He asked me, "Have you been in this house since it's been done over?"

"No, but I'd like to. Dad's had the grand tour."

"I bet he has."

Ted wanted to finish putting up insulation in his basement but he couldn't do it. In the morning, he called Dad and asked him to help him with it. When Dad arrived, he found his son prone on the couch, covered with a blanket, with a fever. That day, Ted was too weak to go for a walk.

Slowing the pace, we approached "our home" on Main Street—Main Street, Kingston, New Hampshire that is. For seventeen years, Teddy and I shared the same bathroom. Constantly, we raced to see who could get there first—one night, he beat me to it.

I slugged down a half a dozen slow gin fizzes, a couple shots of whisky, and I forget what else, trying to drink away my "prissy image" all in one night. As Teddy would say, "I had to take a picked wiss." And, it was my first experience standing in one place watching an entire room spin around me. I was having trouble standing; running was out of the question. As I staggered up the steps, bounced off the doorframe, and slid my shoulder by the coats hanging in the front hall closet—Teddy breezed around me and into the bathroom. I never had a chance.

While he was having a gay old time, peeing to his bladder's content, I stumbled into the kitchen, pinching my thighs together. I could hear Dad coming but there was nowhere to go. I leaned against the tall bureau topped with miscellaneous books, hats, and winter mittens. I held my hand against my temple, with my arm resting on top of a pair of red mittens, and wished the room would stop moving. I wished Teddy would get out of the bathroom so I could go.

"Hi, Dad." My elbow slid off the top of the bureau and one red, hand-knitted mitten landed on the floor. I didn't attempt to bend over to get it.

Dad took one look and decided to leave me alone, "We'll talk about this in the morning."

He was gone before Teddy came sauntering out, "It's all yours."

Nothing was going to stop him—not a doctor, not Brenda, not nobody, not no how! Ted was determined to go to the University of

Maine hockey game with Brenda and Kevin—and he wanted to see Corey. It was November 15, 2003. His blood counts were a disaster (by the end of the week his hemoglobin bottomed out at three and his hematocrit registered as low as nine percent). He went AMA—against medical advice. The brief office visit on that Saturday was enough to get him through the weekend, alive.

Midway through the hockey game Brenda watched as Teddy began to shake.

"Are you okay?" Brenda asked.

"Yeah. I'm okay."

Ted's answer was that he wanted to stay until the end of the game.

I put my kickstand down and leaned against my bike. I glanced up at the second floor, front bedroom where I spent my teenage years. There was no lock on the door. Most often it was left open to the front hall. I was lying on my stomach with my knees bent and my ankles crossed, reading *The Bell Jar*, when I heard footsteps. He was not in a hurry. Teddy ran one hand along the railing. It was shaped in an upside down L, the long side running the length of the upper hallway and the short side running straight to the wallpaper-covered wall. He traced the long side and then followed the short piece into my room. (We used to ride the banister down the long flight of stairs.) I looked up as he came through the door. He was quieter than usual—trying to act like this was a casual visit.

"Whatcha readin'?" He walked across the wooden floor, a few feet into my room, and glanced out the window at The Plains.

"*The Bell Jar*, I have to read it for my English class. Did you have to read it?" I flipped around, pulled my pillow from under the covers, and leaned against the headboard.

"I don't think so. Let me look at it." He stepped away from the window, toward my bed, and reached for the book, "Is it any good?"

"I don't know if I'd call it good, it's kind of upsetting." I pulled my knees up to my chest, and wrapped my arms around them, "Wanna' take a seat?" I nodded to the empty spot at the end of my bed. He sat on my rumpled, yellow puff, thumbing through the pages, not the least bit interested.

"Do you know Tammy Brown?"

I did know Tammy Brown and tried to disguise my disgust. The Tammy Brown I knew was a flirt. She made the rounds and when she was done, she moved on. Tammy was more excited by the hunt than the prey. She was making her move on Ted and I didn't like it. Ted was strong and he was sensitive, but when it came to knowing how to handle females, he wasn't that strong.

"Why do you wanna' know?" I needed time to think.

"I think she likes me."

"What makes you think that?"

"She's been awful chatty around me lately and she keeps staring at me. I think she wants me to ask her out. What do you think of her?"

"I don't really know her very well." As much as I wanted to say, "Run away, Run away," I didn't want to hurt his feelings. "Do you like her?"

"I don't know. She's kind of cute. I guess I like her."

"Do you want to ask her out?"

"I guess so."

"What have you heard about her?"

"I know she just broke up with Bob Darling."

"Anyone else before him?"

"Yeah. I think she went out with Roy Dobbs." He got off my bed and stood for a minute before handing me back my book.

"Do what you want but I'd be careful if I was you." That was about as much as I dared to say.

As he left, he winked over his left shoulder, "Thanks."

Call it mother's intuition. On November 20th, Mom awoke in a fright at 1:00 AM with the strangest feeling. It was unlike any feeling she had ever had before and it tore her apart. She expected the phone to ring and to hear that Teddy was gone. All she wanted to do was get in the car, drive to the hospital, and hug him but that wasn't something she could do. The feeling made her cry until her eyes ached. She wanted him to know that everyone loved him and we wanted him to be at peace. If there is such a thing as extra sensory perception, then I'm sure Ted felt the love that she was sending to him at that moment.

Fifty years before, Mom looked forward to a new baby and prayed it would be a son whom she could watch grow into a man. He had become the man she prayed for and more. Mom was proud of Ted. He was the son, brother, husband, father, uncle, nephew, cousin, and grandson that she hoped he would be. As she slumped over on the kitchen table, with only the light from the full moon to illuminate the darkness around her, tears soaked her flowered nightgown. She loved him so much; how could she let go? She bowed her head, "God bless you, Ted; and Brenda, and Corey, and Kevin."

The next day Mom learned that Ted's hemoglobin and hematocrit counts were extremely low, and that he had had two blood transfusions. His spleen was even larger. The doctors were going back and forth on when and if to take it out. His bone marrow biopsy was not conclusive enough to start another round of chemo. They would have to do another CT scan. Ted was also given news about the second round of testing for a possible sibling donor match.

We glided by the "historical district" row of three Colonial homes; Brenda first, then Jimmy, then Teddy, and then me. Our neighbor's house to the right, closest to the Kingston 1686 House, with the open front porch was empty. The hydrangea bush was not in bloom. The white geraniums in the white, granite urns were fading. The white Colonial to the left of our house stood so close to the road that if anyone stepped out the front door they would step onto the street. That house was still. The rusted hand pump stood unused, marking the corner of their grass-covered yard. To the right of the pump and in between our "middle room" and their glassed-in porch Teddy and Skippy made an igloo.

It had been snowing for three days and school officials finally cancelled school. The snow on the ground piled up ever so close to the edge of our neighbor's barn roof. Teddy and Skippy decided to take a sheet of cardboard and slide off the roof onto the snow bank, before they got yelled at. They dressed in layers—bundled in thermal underwear, ski parkas, woolen hats and mittens, and rubber boots. They kept warm enough to work for hours shoveling snow, piling it high, and carving a hole in the center of a huge mound of pounds of thick, white powder. Kathy and I were inside by the fireplace playing Clue, but every now and then we peeked out the windows. We came out when the igloo was done.

"Can I go in?" Even though I had images of kids playing in igloos and having them cave in, I wanted to see what it was like inside. Teddy smoothed the edges of the hole with his snow-caked mittens, and then finished shaping the entry into the cave. "When I get done." He got on his hands and knees and crawled in while I waited outside. He patted the icy surface on the inside until the rounded walls were packed solid. He poked his head out, "Come on in."

Following his lead, I got on my hands and knees and crawled in. It was dark and it was cold but it wasn't real dark. Light came through the small opening. Though the cave was just big enough to sit up in, I bumped my head on the ceiling. I leaned against the snow curved wall and locked my ankles "Indian style," opposite Teddy. Our boots nearly touched. We were encased in a womb of snow. Not a sound from the outside world could be heard. I sat there imagining what it would be like to be an Eskimo. Teddy must have been thinking about something else, "So, how do you like it?" Ice-cold air smoke escaped from Teddy's mouth. He was pleased with his creation. I was pretty amazed, "This is wicked cool!"

Brenda's message came unexpectedly one evening in November, even though it was anticipated. All along, deep within the recesses of my soul, I felt I would be Teddy's match. I never spoke about it with my siblings. Perhaps, they felt the same. Subconsciously, the feeling that I would be called stayed with me. In the same way I tried to interpret a vivid, powerful dream, I tried to figure out why I felt this way. Yet, it was inexplicable. I heard my cell phone ring and answered the call.

"Guess what, Lucinda?" There was more excitement in Brenda's voice than I had heard in years; she dragged out the moment.

Her excitement triggered my heart rate to race, "I can't guess. What?"

"You're the chosen one." I felt like giving her a high five. She was elated to share the good news and happy it was me. We both were!

I had the same kind of strange feeling that came to Mom in the middle of the night. It was not like any feeling I had ever had before. It was like being wine cooped up in a wine cellar covered in dust, waiting to be properly aged, being carried carefully up a flight of stairs into the Kingston 1686 House reception-filled room, and having the cork popped off. (No blood will spill before it is time.) I called Muffy as soon as I hung up with Brenda. I knew she would understand my jingle, "My blood's better than your blood, my blood's better than yours, my blood's better cause mine matches Ted's...my blood's better than yours!" She got it, and laughed on the other end.

Climbing out of the igloo, there was still plenty of daylight for a snowball fight. Skippy started it. He was hiding behind the white mound waiting for us to come out. Teddy's head and shoulders appeared—like a lion coming out of his wintry den. Skippy beamed him with one strategically-placed snowball, knocking his floppy tassel to one side. Teddy ran for cover by the pump and Kathy and I crouched behind the corner of the house. A huge snowball splattered the back of Kathy's jacket and another one hit me in the leg. We ran from behind the snow-covered pine tree and fought across the yard. We made it to the top of the tallest snow bank, switching from snowballs to hands and fists. We dug our boots into the snow and climbed up the mountain, pushing and shoving each other out of the way. Kathy and I ganged up on Skippy.

With heads down and shoulders tucked, we plowed into him. He fended us off with one hand on each of our heads. While we were spinning out, Teddy knocked Skippy's feet out from under him. Kathy fell, sliding across a patch of ice and I came tumbling after. Skippy landed in a heap of ski parkas on top of us. Teddy was the only one left standing. Covered in snow from his pom-pom tassel to the bottom of his navy-blue, Christmas ski pants, he put both hands on his hips and puffed out his chest. In his best *Wizard of Oz*, Cowardly Lion imitation, he shouted, *if I Were King of the Forest...*

Thanksgiving

Thanksgiving, November 27, 2003, I had lots to be thankful for. My son, my daughter-in-law, and my two grandchildren traveled from Texas to be with us. My daughter, the nurse from New York City, broke away from work and was able to join us. And, the thermostat reached a record fifty-degrees. It was a day to "put the top down" of my convertible.

I let Mandy drive and Matt sat in the front seat. I was content to have the back all to myself. I sat sideways, legs sprawled across the gray velour. I had lived for this moment. We were driving to Kingston for the Thanksgiving morning family football game on The Plains. It was just as exciting now to play football on The Plains as it was thirty-five years ago. The thought still gave me an adrenaline surge. Like a redneck woman I hollered, "Yeah Hah!" as we took off, and shouted instructions to Mandy.

"Mandy, flip the top down. This day is too good to be true. How many Thanksgivings do we get when we can ride with the top down? Put in Shania Twain." This was the first Thanksgiving since Matt went off to college that he had been home for Thanksgiving. Being a nurse, Mandy had to work every other year. This was the first Thanksgiving that I had both my children with me since their high school days. The two of them were not about to give me any grief about my musical selection. Shania was going in.

"You got it, Mom."

As the black top unfolded, a whoosh of warm air caressed us. With the top down I could rest my elbow on the top of the car door. I tipped my head back. My long, loose hair swirled across my eyes, blowing out of control. I was "livin' large." I sang as if I was home alone, *Man! I feel like a woman!* I pounded to the beat on Matt's shoulders and kept on keeping on. Matt and Mandy grinned at each other. Their eyes said, "Yup, she's lost it." I was thinking, "It doesn't get any better than this."

From *I'm Holding On To Love* to *Don't Be Stupid*, Shania and I belted our way to Kingston. I was back in the old days. I was fifteen. Brenda and I were riding with Pat and a best friend by the name of Steve. Steve, "Frap Man," was beating on the car we all envied. I was in the back seat of his GTO watching him finger his steering wheel as if it was his guitar; and hitting his dashboard drum. The words, the beat, the volume had a power that moved through him. It was the same for me. This power started in my churned-up belly and forced its way out of me. I was a wolf howling at the moon. I was Teddy and Pat jumping off a tall bridge—standing anxiously on the edge of the struts, letting out a breath, and leaping to the running water below. I was a giddy teenage girl. This "let it all hang-out" behavior was a knee-jerk reaction to stimulation in life that ignored inhibitive norms. It was doing something because the power to move spoke louder than the power to stay put. I listened to Shania and sang into the wind, the car was getting me where I wanted to go but something else drove me.

When I saw the crowd of relatives already gathered on The Plains I told Mandy to honk the horn, and yelled to Matt, "Fast forward it to my favorite song and turn it up louder!" Mandy pulled down the side street and parked beside the ditch. Shania swooned, "Honey, I'm Home!" I jumped out of the car, skipped over the ditch and ran toward Skippy raising my right arm and waving, "Pass it to me, pass it to me!"

Skippy fondled the football, twirling it in his hands as he looked my way, and nodded his head. He heaved it into the air. I watched its projection carefully and anticipated its arrival, noting the hole in the ground to my right. I hopped over the hole, opening both arms. Man, I felt like a woman, as the pointed end of the pigskin dug into my right boob. I had forgotten how hard a regulation football is but I was glad that I hadn't lost my touch. I called out, "Can't we play with a nerf ball?"

A whole bunch of us—sisters, brothers, aunts, uncles, cousins, etc. were milling around. It was time to choose sides. Once again, Dad would have to settle for ref. Muffy and I hip-checked each other and started talking trash.

"I'm gonna be the quarterback…"

"Yeah, well I'm gonna be the center."

"Momma's gonna knock you out…"

"I'm gonna quarterback sneak and watch you land on your butt…"

"Oh yeah…"

"Yeah…"

We jumped up and down shouting to the captains, Ronnie (my nephew) and Skippy, "Pick me, Pick me!"

All this running around and jumping up and down made me spill some urine. Birthing a ten-pound baby caused that little problem. I stopped jumping and concentrated on getting on a team.

It doesn't matter how old you are, you still want to be picked. I was relieved when Skippy pointed his finger at me. I joined his yakking group of rag-tag hooligans; sticking my tongue out at Muffy. My captain, my captain called us into a huddle, "All right, everyone block except Bryan. Bryan you go long and I'll hit you in the left pocket." Muffy's pudgy nose and my longer nose were tip to tip. I taunted her, "You're goin' down, kid."

She wiggled her butt and scrunched her nose up at me, "Who you callin' kid?"

Getting ready to shove her off, I retorted, "Oh yeah, I almost forgot…you are a lot older than me."

I pushed her aside watching Jimmy escaping around the end; running straight for my quarterback. Skippy, still fit at fifty, dodged to the right in time to get the ball out of his hands. It spun through the air on its way to Bryan, Skippy's son; and my niece, Emily, was hot on his trail. Bryan was across the end zone—the imaginary line before the ditch—when he managed to catch the ball and hold it tight. Trying to dodge Emily, he arched his back. She was pretty fast. She is actually pretty…and a fast runner. She tagged Bryan with both hands. We made it clear—touch, not tackle.

"Touchdown!" I yelled, slapping Skippy across his shoulder.

"Emily got him," Muffy sneered at me.

"He was clearly in the end zone." I put my hands on my hips and turned to Dad.

"What's the call, Dad?"

Dad raised both his arms into the air, "Touchdown!" We didn't argue with him, and went to huddle-up.

Ronnie, towering over Jimmy, put his arm around his neck and whispered in his ear. I suspected he was trying to pull a razzle-dazzle play out of his semi-professional days. Though he was grinning, football for all of us was serious business. At thirty-something, with his six pack abs, he could show us all a thing or two. I snuck across the field and put my ear through a space between Emily and Jordan. "She's cheatin', she's cheatin'." I ran back to my own huddle, unashamed.

I told Skippy, "Watch out, he's gonna try somethin' tricky."

"All right, Cin, we'll be ready. Bryan, you cover Jimmy and I'll watch out for Jordan. They might try to lateral back to the little guy."

We lined up. I stared at Jordan, with his wiry, boyish frame, and sang him a familiar rhyme, "Jordan is a friend of mine, he resembles Frankenstein, when he does the Irish jig, he resembles Porky Pig." He gave me a poker face, ignoring my diversionary tactic. Ronnie started the play, "Hut one, hut two, hut three."

Emily and Mandy spread out in a V, while Jimmy stepped over the scrimmage line. Muffy, close to the ground, scrambled to block Bryan; Tyler, not concerned with the play, whipped his sister to the ground; Jeff, an ex-Richmond College Spider, cleared the way for me; and I rushed the quarterback. I didn't want them to score. Running straight for him, I ducked my head and locked my arms. "What was I thinking?" Ronnie saw me coming and as he threw Jimmy the ball, braced himself. I collided into his chest, as he brought his arms up in a defensive posture. When he raised his arms he clipped my chin with the back of his knuckles and I fell back, landing on solid turf. He cut me down. I caved like a tiny sapling. For sure, my teeth were rattled. Dazed, I moved my jaw to the right and then to the left hoping it wasn't broken. It took me a minute to get off the ground. I felt a drop of blood oozing from the split under my chin, and thought to myself, "Now, I'm in trouble. Pat told me not to get carried away."

Ronnie looked at me confused, "Are you all right?"

"Look, what you've done to your poor aunt." I lifted my chin so he could get a closer look. It was scraped and bruised.

"I'm sorry."

"You ought to be, you big brute."

"I'm sorry."

"We should have an automatic touchdown for that."

"I'm not that sorry."

We laughed it off and returned to our respective huddles. I wasn't the only one to get hurt that day. Poor Jordan, one of the youngest guys out there, got plowed over like a decayed corn stalk in Uncle Harry's field.

I played for a little while longer, but the hit shook me up pretty good. Before I could get myself hurt again, I took my pride and my bruised chin, and slunk to the sidelines. My play wasn't as dramatic as Teddy taking a bite out of John's head but I had a good story to tell him later. Ashton, my three-year-old granddaughter, had come to the field and it was time for me to act like a grandmother—whatever that means. Kathy was there with her two daughters. I heard they wanted a ride in my convertible. I was more than happy to give them the "Shania Twain" special, whether they liked her music or not. As Shania says, "In my car...I am the driver," which is another excellent tune to beat on the dashboard.

I woke up the next morning feeling the stiffness in my jaw, but was grateful that it wasn't broken and no teeth were missing. My family was all around me but the tide-like pull to see Ted was strong. I knew he wasn't doing well. He missed the football game and God only knows what kind of Thanksgiving he had had. Pat felt the pull as well.

"What do you want to do today?" He asked with apprehension.

"I want to see Teddy." There was no question in my mind.

"I know he wanted that insulation put up in his basement that he's been trying to get to."

"I know. Maybe, we can do that for him."

We called Becky's husband, Ron. He and his son, Jeff, wanted to go too. The four of us piled in the Explorer and drove to Loudon. When we got there the house was quiet. Brenda greeted us at the door.

"Thanks for comin'. Teddy's sleepin' in his chair."

I looked at the chair, the black leather recliner and drew in a breath. Ted's head was resting against the pillow. Hair stubble covered his chin. His mouth was slightly open, but there was no drool. He was too dry for that. A thick blanket was pulled up around his neck. His skin was deathly pale. I had all I could do not to gasp out loud. When he heard our noises his eyes flickered open. A frail voice came from deep within, "Heyyyyy, CC," he paused, "Thanks for comin'." He didn't try to get up. I wanted to cry.

I walked over to his chair, bent down, and kissed him on the cheek, "I love you," I said softly.

He looked me in the eyes and repeated, "I love you too."

"I hear we have some work to do."

"Yeah, the man of the house has taken some time off."

"It figures. He always was a lazy cuss."

"The stuff's all in the basement, I'm sure Pat can figure it out."

"You think so?" I asked, but we both knew Pat could handle the job. I followed Brenda into the kitchen and let the guys talk to him. She filled me in.

"He's had fevers again and keeps shaking. He's real short of breath. I'm waiting to get in touch with his doctor."

"Brenda, how are you?"

"I'm fine."

It was just as difficult to get her to spill her guts as it was Teddy. In some ways, they were two of a pair—maybe, too much so. She led us into the basement. One would think it was a bomb shelter waiting for an air raid. There were shelves and shelves of mustard, ketchup, and other non-perishables.

"Why all the mustard, Brenda?" I couldn't help but ask.

"We order from this food company and it's a good deal."

"It's a good deal but isn't it going to take you forever to use it all up?"

She laughed, "It will get used eventually."

"Whatever you say. I know where I can get some ketchup if I ever get desperate."

She walked us toward the end of the basement and showed us where Teddy had left off, and then she started back up the stairs. On the third step she turned and looked back, "I can get you lunch later if you want." We each offered her our, "No thanks." None of us had much of an appetite.

We lifted boards and brushed away saw dust looking around for duct tape, a staple-gun, and cutters to break up the insulation. I looked across the basement ceiling and saw the open bays. Our task was to fill the openings with sheets of insulation. Jeff and I paired up, while Pat and Ron started "calculating the square root of an isosceles triangle." They were summing up the situation. Jeff pulled a ladder over near the stairs. I waited for a piece of insulation to poke up in to the foot-wide space, "He does not look good. I am so worried."

Jeff put his head down, "I know," and continued working "Pat, could you hand me the staple-gun?"

Pat found it on the work-bench and handed it over, "I think we should measure a few first," he said. Pat wanted to make sure there was enough material to get us through the project.

The whole time we worked in the basement, I felt the weight from above. It was so heavy, at times, I had trouble breathing. The image of Ted in the chair followed me down the stairs. It haunted all my thoughts. I wondered if he would make it through this day. How did he live through last weekend? I began to think of him as the walking dead man.

"Did you see how pale he was?" I asked no one in particular. No one chose to respond. Now, if I were in the basement with my sisters the conversation would have been very different. For one thing, there would have been a lot more whispering about what we should do. There would have been speculation about what was going on. Muffy would have had a hard time being quiet and so would Becky. Becky would have taken his blood pressure, and Muffy would have pumped him for information. But then, I was with men, and men don't go around wondering about the "what if's." Like a blind man who picked up his hammer and saw, men "see" through their work. It's no wonder Pat, Ron, Jeff, and Ted all liked Conan so much. He was a doer. For forty days and forty nights (at least that's what I say) he turned the wheel under the blazing sun and got stronger for it. Conan didn't sit around discussing his fate. In fact, he didn't talk much at all.

Being busy was helpful but I felt so useless. How could I sit by and see him suffer so? Wasn't there something that could be done for him? When would he get to the doctor? I wanted to go upstairs, but what good would that do? I pushed up on the insulation and reached for some duct tape to cover the space between the insulation and the beam. I looked down at Jeff, "Ted wouldn't want any gaposis."

He smiled and handed me the next piece. We worked our way to the end of that bay and then I climbed down the ladder, ready to do the next section. Brenda's running sneakers, then her jeans, then her tan sweater, then her hunched shoulders, then her streaked hair, then her face… showing signs of despair; appeared in the stairway.

Her eyes darted from the cement floor to eye level, never stopping to focus, "Ted has an appointment at the hospital at 2:00."

"Do you need any help getting him in the car?"

"No, that's okay, Kevin can help me." As quickly as she had come, she was gone.

I looked at my watch noting the time. It would be another hour. In slow motion, step by step, I left the three men without saying a word and went to my brother. I passed the wood stove, the tall glass windows, the round kitchen table, and then the oval dining room table. I could see the back of his yellow baseball hat motionless against the soft leather. I walked around to the side of his chair and knelt down. His eyes were closed but he felt my presence and he opened them, "How's it goin' down there?"

I gave him a snapshot, "Pat and Ron have figured it all out. Jeff and I are doin' the grunt work. We're gettin' there." Then, I needed to ask, "How are you?" His chin began to tremble and one tear leaked from the corner of his left eye, and drifted down his cheek. A single tear told me his story. In a muffled voice, his words were difficult to hear, but easy to understand, "Not so good."

I came halfway up to standing and crouched over him, the puffy arm of his chair getting in my way. I reached around his sweaty, thin back and tried to pull him close. He lifted his left arm from under his blanket and responded to my touch. The brim of his hat bopped my forehead and came partly off his head. In the hugging, he must have glimpsed my pinkish scars, "What happened to your chin?" I released my hold, "I got that playing football yesterday. Ronnie clobbered me." Faintly, he smiled, "I hope you got the best of him."

"Not really," I confessed. "I wish you could have been there. I could have used your help." With that, I slipped away to the bathroom and grabbed a few tissues before returning to the basement.

Piece by piece, the insulation was cut to size, the ladder moved across the floor, and staples locked the insulation into place. Idle chatter got us from bay to bay.

"So, Jeff, how's your job goin'?"

"It's going good. I'm liking it for now."

I heard footsteps move across the floor up above and a door squeak open.

"Do you think you'll ever move up here to New Hampshire?"

"I don't know. Maybe. It depends on the job."

I heard a car door slam.

"Do you still watch Conan on Christmas eve?"

"When I can. It's tradition."

I heard the car back out of the driveway.

Christmas

I learned the next day, through a conversation with Mom, that Teddy was seen at the hospital and sent home. I couldn't believe it. All they did was draw some blood and instruct him to come back the next day. I woke up expecting to hear that he had been admitted. I tried to imagine what kind of night Brenda and Teddy had. It scared me to think of his breathing, his color, and his severe weakness. How did he make it through the night? On Saturday, as instructed, he went back to Concord Hospital where he was given three units of blood and one unit of platelets. I silently gave a huge thank you to all those people who faithfully give blood. Without it, Ted would have been dead by now. Mom informed me, "He was still weak, but doing better." In the meantime, the plan was to continue with more chemotherapy and prepare for an allogeneic stem cell transplant.

Subject: Ted
From: Jim Clark
Date: Tue, 2 Dec 2003
Hello all,
Update on Ted:

- *Ted met with doctor today and is at home*
- *Chemo next Tuesday 12/09/03 (either Concord or Dartmouth)*
- *Anyone wishing to visit Ted must have a flu shot.*
- *Stay away from Ted if you have any cold like symptoms*
- *Thoughts and well wishes to Ted always welcome!!*

Muffy gleefully replied to all, "Hi, Ted, Guess which sister has already had her flu shot and can see you? It's not Lucinda (aka Cindy) and it's not Becky, Debby, or Dolly. You guessed it! The smart one. Muffy."

(I had to hand it to her for that one, as the emails continued.)

> *Subject: Ted*
> *From: Jim Clark*
> *Date: Sun, 7 Dec. 2003*
> *Hello all,*
> *Enjoying all the snow? I could have gone to Pat's game today, but said no. I hate the traffic. Spoke to Ted yesterday. Here is the latest:*
>
> - *Ted sounded great!*
> - *He and Brenda toured their land in Franconia after paying taxes.*
> - *His blood counts were up slightly.*
> - *He will attend a support group Tuesday (great idea)*
> - *He will have chemo treatment Wednesday now at Concord.*
> - *I got Ted the latest Lance Armstrong book (Every Second Counts) but need to get it to him. I have not had a flu shot yet so I can't give it to him. Who can drop it off for me? By the way this is an excellent book and enjoyable reading even if you don't like cycling.*

My secret fear for Ted was that he was busy trying to please his family, yet, I wasn't quite sure what pleased him. Did he want to talk about his cancer? Did he want to hear about other experiences of cancer patients? What gave him the most comfort? Did he feel better talking to cancer survivors…or did it make him feel worse? If they lived to tell about it and he did not, would that make him a failure in his eyes? Would he feel guilty for not willing himself to get better? I had seen the spiritual self-help books at his bedside, and on his coffee table. My suspicion came from a few fleeting words during one of my visits. He looked at me in distress, "What if I'm not being positive enough?" My fear was confirmed. I tried to mitigate its meaning. I said what I thought was right to say, "Ted, Abigail Philips was one of the most positive people I've ever known. She was spiritual. She was strong. She was a fighter. Somehow, she managed to be uplifting to others, in spite of her cancer. She died. Not everyone can be Lance Armstrong. Not everyone can will themselves to get better. Please, do not feel guilty for whatever it is you are feeling. You have a right to feel the way you do."

It was my only conversation with him about the subject. It was never brought up again. It was short and it was sweet, but it wasn't real sweet.

While Teddy was busy having chemo, I had my own very minor medical affliction and phobia. A fear is a fear and sometimes no matter how hard you try to make it less so, you cannot get it out of your head. Or, in my case, out of my ears. I'm convinced that everyone has some kind of phobia. It might be the dentist. It might be staying alone at night. It might be driving over a bridge. Teddy confided in me one time that he couldn't stand the thought of someone having a sharp object go through his leg and split it open. He had seen it happen in a skiing accident when he was on ski patrol. He shuddered telling me about it. With me it's having wax removed from my ears. No matter how much I try to will myself that there is nothing to it, there always is. I think it's the fear of having a sharp object puncture my eardrum and how painful that would be.

This December, I waited so long to go to the doctor that I became deaf in my left ear. Popping it just wouldn't clear it any longer. I got tired of answering the phone with my right ear and finally made the appointment. My ENT doctor prescribed Ativan to get me through it.

Calmly and professionally, he told me what to do, "Fill the prescription before you come to the office. Then, take the pill in the waiting room and wait about twenty minutes. You should be all set when we call you in."

I drove to Rite Aid and went to the counter. It felt as if the pharmacist handed me a bag of air; I looked inside to make sure something was there. A tiny orange container with a white label rested inside. I reached in, pulled it out, and held it up to the light. One itsy bitsy pill rolled along the bottom of the bottle not making a sound. It was no bigger than an eraser tip on a number two pencil. I thought, "I hope this does the trick," and held the bag tightly as I proceeded to the empty waiting room. I took my tiny, little pill in private and chose a chair that was back-to to the reception desk, and then let my mind wander. Like Teddy's deep-sea fishing trip, this excursion would prove to be a sickening experience.

"Hey, Boris, you wanna' go deep-sea fishin'?" Pat asked him.

"Sure, when you goin'?"

"Next weekend. A bunch of us are goin' out on Eastman's boat."

"That's out of Seabrook, right?"

"Yeah, it's on the Seabrook side of Hampton harbor, right near the Hampton bridge."

"What kind of fish?"

"Mostly cod and haddock."

I began to feel a little sleepy and light in the head. A middle-aged man about five feet eleven inches tall took a seat near me, and I glanced his way. I smiled but I didn't attempt a conversation. Maybe this pill was going to work after all.

"It might get a little rough out there today," the captain warned.

"No problem for us, right, Ted?"

Ted lifted his right eyebrow and gave his buddy Pat a questioning stare. He wasn't so sure about that. I doubt he popped a Dramamine—another very small pill. That would involve planning. Clouds covered most of the sky as he tromped up the silvery, metal ramp onto the boat. A squawking seagull splattered the edge of the fiberglass with loose green and white shit, which slid into the salty water. The forty-two foot, diesel-powered "party boat" kept bobbing in the surf as the captain's mate mumbled his instructions. A wiry, seventeen-year-old, with long, windswept, dirty blond hair repeated the familiar drill, "Give a holla' when you need more chum and I'll get it to yeah. Holla' if yeah need any help. We have plenty of extra hooks to bring in the big ones."

"Lucinda Marcoux," the nurse called my name and I followed her down the hall. She held the door with her right hand and motioned with her left. She directed me in to the second office on the left and asked, "How are you?"

"I'm okay, but I think I'm beginning to feel a little dizzy."

"Did you take the Ativan?"

"Yes I did."

"That should help. Just take a seat and the doctor will be right in." She left my chart on his desk on the way out the door. I climbed into the dentist-like chair and laid my head against the back, closing my eyes.

There was more than gentle rolling as Eastman's fishing boat entered deeper water. The shore was out of sight and all that was visible was the sky, the water, and the waves that kept coming, and coming, and coming. As Teddy baited his fishing line and flung it out to sea, he knocked over the metal bucket at his foot, forcing him to spread his legs to keep his balance. The boat sunk deeper in the water and then quickly rose. Teddy felt every motion of the ocean like riding an elevator to the fourteenth floor and having it stop on the fifth, the eighth, the eleventh, and finally the fourteenth, only this elevator wasn't ever going to stop.

I heard the door open and saw Dr. Sim's short, unassuming shape saunter toward my left side. Smiling he asked, "How are you today?"

"Well, considering how much I enjoy this procedure, I'm doin' just fine."

Dr. Sim was well acquainted with my neurosis and seemed to take it in stride. He'd seen me at my worst. The first time I met "the man" he had to send me to a local pharmacy for Ativan, midway through the session. I thought he was the most patient man I had ever met. It was love at first ear-wax removal. He picked up his flashlight and gently searched my ear, "Yup, this one's pretty blocked. Let's take a look in the other one."

"The other one is fine," I assured him, "it's always my left one."

"You're right. Let's get started."

"Could your nurse hold my hand?" Embarrassed as I was...I had to ask.

He smiled again, turned away from me, and went out the door to find his nurse.

"I think I got one, Boris, come give me a hand." Pat was pulling back on his pole, leaning toward the edge of the glassed-in cabin.

"I'm comin'." Teddy pulled in his line, let his pole drop to the wave-soaked floor, and skidded his way over to Pat. He grabbed the lower end of the pole and together they pulled as hard as they could. They pulled back, and bent forward; pulled back, and bent forward; pulled back, and bent forward. Just as they thought they were going to pull the big fish out of the water, Teddy let go of his grip.

Dr. Sim returned with his nurse and set up his equipment, some kind of suctioning tool and a basin for the wax. As he tenderly tugged at my earlobe and started suctioning out the wax, I gripped my nurse's hand.

"Does it hurt?" He sounded genuinely concerned.

I wanted to lie and be done with this, but I told the truth, "It doesn't really hurt, I just hate the sensation."

"We can stop." I couldn't believe he was giving me this option.

"No. I'm all right, just keep goin'." I uncurled my toes, listening to the loud whirring of an obscure sucking machine as it probed the inside of my left ear.

"Well, let me know if you need me to stop." He patted me on the shoulder and continued.

As the boat swayed to the right, Teddy ran for the railing. He leaned his chest against the fiberglass and pitched forward, hurling pink and green chunks over the side. Squiggly tips of white water crashed against the navy blue letters of Eastman's Charter Cruises, as Teddy's vomit hit in waves.

"You need some help, Boris?" Pat put down his pole and walked toward him, forgetting about the fish that got away.

Teddy wobbled, his knees buckling, as he groped his way to a chair. He slumped down; elbows on his knees and hands bracing his head, any trace of fresh-air redness disappearing from his face. A pair of pliers slid across the slimy wood and clinked against the metal bucket.

"You gonna be all right, Boris?" Pat knew he was done for.

Teddy raised his head slightly and grinned, "Didn't you say you needed some more chum?"

When Dr. Sim could see clear to my eardrum he stopped, "Looks like we got it all. You should be able to hear a lot better now. Why don't you book your appointments more frequently so it doesn't get quite so bad?"

"It takes me six months to build up my nerve to come. You think I'm gonna make it in more often?"

Again, he smiled and wished me well as he left the room. Pitifully, as if Oliver Twist, I turned to his nurse and asked for one more favor, "Please miss, may I have a glass of cold water?" By now the Ativan was starting to take over, and I felt a bit woozy, and I needed to sit there for a few minutes to get composed.

The nurse handed me my water, "Are you all right?"

"I think so. I just need a few more minutes."

"Well, take your time and you can leave when you're ready." She left me alone—probably relieved to get to another patient.

"Thank you so much." I sat until I thought I was okay.

I didn't realize how drastically the Ativan had begun to affect me until I started driving to work. The more I tried to concentrate, the harder it became. The white line in the center of the road kept moving. It was as if I were three months pregnant trying to drive to work through a steady, but light mesmerizing snow. Rolling the window down and pinching my thigh didn't help. I could not keep my eyes open, and had to pull off the side of the road. I found myself pulling into the parking lot of DeMoula's grocery store.

I veered into the parking lot near the corner of the building and stopped with the engine still running. My head was resting against my driver-side windshield when I heard rapping. I rolled my window down to a man I had never seen before.

"Miss, are you all right?"

"Yeah, I was just at the doctor's."

"You better pull into a parking spot."

I tried to make sense out of what he was saying, managing to recognize that I was stopped in the middle of the parking lot. I said, "Thank you."

He appeared out of nowhere then he was gone. He disappeared into the foggy landscape of my Ativan-created world. I did as he told me and drove my car into the nearest empty spot, fortunate that I didn't hit anyone or anything. I was in a deep sleep when I heard the next rap at my window—a police officer. She kindly asked me to roll down my window.

"Miss, could I see your license?"

I struggled to sit up straight. I fished through my pocketbook and handed her my wallet showing her my picture, "What's wrong?"

"You seem to be having a little trouble here. Is there someone I could call to come get you?"

"I guess I had a reaction to some medication I just took. My dad works at the East Kingston Town Hall. He could probably come and get me."

While the concerned police officer went back to her car to look up the number for the East Kingston Town Hall, I flipped my head back against the car door. I was conscious long enough to hope that my dad could be reached. Yet, I was not conscious enough to move, and promptly drifted back to sleep. When Teddy slept in his hospital bed he opened his eyes to family members staring at him—it was disorienting. I was disoriented, too, when I heard the next rapping at my car window.

"Cindy, are you okay?" Dad asked.

"I guess so. I guess I'm kind of out of it."

"Well, I've come to drive you home."

"What about my car?"

"Jimmy will come back for that later."

I looped my fingers around the straps of my pocketbook, collected my rubbery legs, and leaned out of the car. As if I had just ridden on the "round-up" at the 4th of July Kingston Carnival, I bent over the tar and vomited. It splattered the tar. I straightened up just enough to walk the five feet to my dad's car and lowered myself into the front seat. I wanted Scottie to beam me up, but my dad's Ford Escort was a good substitute—I didn't remember getting from DeMoula's to my driveway.

Once I found my puffy red living room couch, there was no getting up again. I slept the rest of the afternoon. This time it was rapping at my dining room door that woke me up. It was Mom.

"How are you feeling?"

"A lot better. I still feel kind of weird, but I am better. I can't believe what that little pill did to me. I'll never take that again."

As Mom worried about her son, she never lost sight of events happening throughout the world, writing daily entries in her diary. She filled it with information about Ted's condition and interspersed it with things like, "Sadaam Hussein was captured today." The date was Sunday, December 14, 2003.

She was always concerned for those who were less fortunate. She taught us to feel blessed for what we had. Her capacity to put things into perspective was, no doubt, part of her strength and what sustained her through the tougher days. She never asked, "Why Teddy?" She said with conviction, "Teddy has had such a good life," or "Think about the ones that don't have any family," or "What if he didn't have any insurance?" or "At least he has great medical care." Mom didn't send her son off to fight in Iraq, yet, she watched cancer wage a war against Ted's body that was fought with one battle after another. Still, as bad as it got, she knew it could be worse.

Mom, Dad, Becky, Ron, Ronnie, Pat and I were determined to get to the Verizon Center in Manchester, New Hampshire for the UNH versus Dartmouth basketball game. We all wanted to see Dave's team play in this new venue. A Nor'easter was predicted. It was overcast, but it wasn't snowing when we started out—by the time we hit Route 101 snow was beginning to accumulate. Pat switched on the windshield wipers. As we merged onto Route 286, a fast-moving Subaru slid sideways without stopping, slowing to forty-miles per hour. It was a wake-up call. Visibility was cut in half with each gust of wind, but it didn't rattle Pat. He was an excellent driver. After snow storms, Pat, Ted, and Skippy did "doughnuts" in the school parking lot while I held onto the door handle. It prepared them on how to handle all kinds of weather conditions and taught me how to "go along for the ride."

Mom, and the rest of us, tried to read between the slanted lines of snow, on signs directing us to the Verizon Center. It became a challenge, especially in the dark. Turning on to Bridge Street, our winter wiper blades kept a steady pace with the mounting flecks of white snow, but heavy precipitation was starting to form along the outside edges of the glass. In a "candid photo op" we were framed inside the crusty, front windshield of the moving vehicle. I kept wondering if Teddy and Brenda were going to make it.

Pat maneuvered alongside the sidewalk in front of the main entrance. "You guys get out and I'll go find a place to park," he said.

"Do you want me to come with you?" I asked from the back, but Ron had already decided to stay with him and wasn't getting out.

"Just go get the tickets and we'll be in as soon as we can."

I pulled up my suede fur-lined hood and raised my arm to shield my face against the wind as I headed for the huge, glass doors, squinting to see my way. Bundled-up bodies moved in a cluster, hunched over on their way to the brick-faced building. Nobody bothered to look up. I was glad I wore my knee-high, rubber-soled, Kittery Trading Post, tan suede boots as I sank into four inches of snow on the sidewalk. The short distance from the road to the building was enough to coat us in white.

Mom and I were inside, stomping our boots on the cold cement and shaking off the snow when she asked, "Do you think Teddy and Brenda will still try to come?"

"I hope not. But, then again, they probably will."

We bought our tickets and meandered through the halls, looking for the way to the gym. It was eerie, standing at the top of the bleachers, looking out over an empty court. The two teams hadn't come out yet to practice. The padded players' chairs were lined-up neatly to the left and right of the scorers' table. The white nylon nets were suspended in the air—open pillow cases waiting to get stuffed. The scoreboard that records the story was black. There were no bells, no whistles, and no sounds of dribbling. The emptiness of such a large, enclosed room and the anticipation of a difficult game ahead, coming at the tail-end of a trying season, made me feel hollow. It was a season filled with the usual ups and downs, but this season… there were more downs than ups. Only the most devoted, or crazy, spectators would bother to come out on a night like this. Slowly, fans trickled in and sat wherever they pleased. We chose the middle of the west side of the stadium seating. Taking my seat, I looked over my left shoulder searching for Ted.

The game started with the introduction of coaches and players, the shaking of hands in the middle of the circle, and the jump ball. It was before Ted and Brenda arrived. Although they had driven in a snow storm, their tardiness was not what made this remarkable. They often tended to be late. "Foul!" I heard the shrill of the ref's whistle as Ted appeared at the railing. He looked down over the Clark clan and began to negotiate his descent.

The walking dead man, as pale as Boo Radley, smiled when our eyes met, making a connection. I left my seat and went to greet him. He stood with his hands stuffed in his pockets, tipping a bit from side to side, as I approached.

"Hey, CC," he drawled.

"Hey, Ted. I'm glad you could make it. How was the drivin'?"

"Not bad."

"Yeah, right." I knew he didn't want to make an issue of it, so I let it go. "Let's go sit down." I felt, right or wrong, that he needed to get off his feet.

We slid in next to Ron and Pat, and continued our conversation. He glanced at the court, "So, how's it goin'?"

"Not so good. UNH is up by six."

He looked at Dave who was wiping his forehead, "Dave'll get on 'em."

"Yup. He will. I hope they can come up with a W."

"Me, too."

Looking away from the court, I asked, "What have you been up to?"

"Went to Kevin's soccer game Friday night."

"Indoor soccer, huh?"

"Yeah. It' pretty neat."

"How did Kevin do?"

"He did pretty well."

"Probably better than you, I think you confused soccer with football."

He grinned as he asked, "What's new with you?"

"Well...I created quite a stir the other day."

Puzzled, he asked, "How's that?"

"You know how I hate to have my ears messed with. Right?"

"I guess so." He actually hadn't heard the extent of my phobia.

I filled him in on my recent trip to the doctor.

He smiled, "That's too much." He paused, "I take Ativan."

"You do?"

"Yeah, it helps me with my nerves."

"Well, it might have helped me get through the wax removal, but I'll never take it again."

"It works for me."

Dartmouth fans erupted as the "Big Green" hit a three-pointer and our focus went back to the game. Everyone was clapping as I thought…about Ativan. So, this is what it has come to. My big brother is taking a medication to help him relax. The stress of his illness has to be pretty bad. I was glad to know there was something that could give him some relief.

As a blue-and-white uniformed six-footer pulled up for an easy lay-up in the paint, I wondered how much snow was piling up outside. The driving was probably going to be worse going home than it was getting here. I elbowed Pat, "Do you think we should leave before the end of the game?" He shook his head, "No." I stayed put in my uncomfortable seat, worried about Dartmouth losing, worried about us getting home safe, and worried about Ted. What if they get in an accident? By the time the deafening buzzer finally sounded the end of the game, I had stored up enough worry to bounce ME off the walls. I wanted to know who was going to drive home—Ted or Brenda. I pulled Brenda aside and asked, "Are you going to do the driving?" She frowned and said, "Ted wants to drive." I kept my mouth shut and started worrying some more.

In small clusters, fans filed out of the gym, zipping up jackets and putting on gloves. I pulled my hood up, braced for the cold blast of frigid air, and pushed the glass door with my shoulder. I looked toward the street. One brightly-lit street light illuminated a parked car. Two silhouettes in the night huddled over, trying to deflect the onslaught of steady, accumulating snow. They bolted, making holes in the drifts, for their car. Weightless, white drops whirled in the air and circled around my curved hood. Some of them managed to reach my cheeks. They melted on contact.

"Wait inside until I pull up the car," Pat instructed.

I turned against the crowd and snuck back inside. Wrapped in a swarm of exiting spectators, Ted and Brenda were about to leave the building. I was able to get close enough to utter my parting words, "Please…be careful driving home." It was probably a stupid thing to say; like he wasn't going to be careful on this white-out producing, inevitable skidding, and nerve-testing night! But, I had to say it anyway. A sliver of a smile crept across his face, and then faded as he stepped out the door.

Ted moved with the same sense of mission as my daughter as she tromped alone across the unplowed parking lot in back of her school's gym in semi-darkness. I watched her with the same heavy heart that I watched Ted. They both carried burdens that I could not help them with. Though I wanted to ease their pain, nothing I could do or say seemed to help. To everything there is a season—a time to hold on, a time to let go. As excruciating as it is, as a mother… or as a sister, you learn to know the difference. Sometimes, they have to fight their own battles. You can be with them in spirit, but they have to go it alone.

Bodies leaned against the wind and quickly spread out in a contrived formation like a reverse constellation of black stars against a sky of white. Teddy was one of many in the crowd but his movement was in contrast to the others. His steps were slow, deliberate, and labored. His winter jacket didn't fit him very well. Gusts of wind made it puff out from his thin waistline. Ted's yellow baseball hat was more ornamental than protective. It was no match for *Glamdring, the foe hammer*, or this winter weather. He hunched his shoulders and kept his hands in his pockets, lifting one heavy foot and then the other. His baggy pants flapped in the wind, as snow swirled from his head to his toes. He stopped at the intersection and waited for the lights to change. The energy of the street lamp cast a mist of light over the shadow of his figure. I watched him look both ways and cross the street, then disappear into the abyss of this niveous night—until he was out of reach.

Subject: Ted
From: Jim Clark
Date: Tue, 23 Dec 2003
Update on Ted:
Ted and Brenda went to Dartmouth. Left early AM and gone until 7:30 tonight.

- *IV was put in to give Ted more blood and platelets to boost counts*

- *Also IV put in to give Ted morphine to help ease some pain while having 2 bone marrow biopsies*
- *Unfortunately IV began to leak under skin and could not be used for chemo. They tried different times to insert new IV to administer the needed chemotherapy.*
- *Doctor even tried in Ted's neck to no avail*
- *Ted will go again to Dartmouth (7:00 AM) to have a pic line inserted or hopefully be able to get just an IV line, for chemo treatment.*
- *Real good news: the results of PET Scan showed no lit up areas (white) anywhere, even in spleen.*
- *Spleen has shrunk.*
- *Looks like Cindy (go girl!) is the one!! Either she will donate bone marrow or may donate stem cells peripherally.*
- *No result from CAT Scan yet.*
- *Waiting result of bone marrow biopsy.*

Ted has had 2 long days and 1 more tomorrow. Hopefully he will get some rest for X-mas. He sounded real good. May this be a X-mas for healing.

Love to all this X-mas,
Jim

    When I got the note, all I could think about was what his Christmas day would be like. I knew Ted would be lucky to be at home with his family, and not in the hospital. With the holiday approaching, and Ted's Christmases appearing to be numbered, I thought a lot about Christmases we had shared.

    I was thirteen when Teddy came home from Christmas shopping—looking like the Cheshire cat. He was a grin without a body. He was so excited about his purchases; he could not wait for Christmas—literally, he could not wait for Christmas. I heard the familiar rustling sound of a large, brown paper bag. His fist was wrapped tightly over the edges of the bag while he waved it in front of my face.

    "You wanna' see what I got you for Christmas?" He teased.

    "No. I want to wait. Don't show it to me now."

    "I'm gonna give it to you now." He started to release his fist.

    "Come on. Wait until Christmas."

"Nope. Not gonna." He peeled the bag open and looked inside.

I closed my eyes, "I don't want to see it." I started laughing as he tickled my neck with the edge of the bag.

"CC. Open your eyes." He was scolding me.

I put my hands over my eyes, "Leave me alone." I laughed some more knowing he wasn't going to give up.

"But it's really cool. You're gonna like it." He shook the bag and reached to pull my hands away from my eyes.

"All right. All right. I give in." I couldn't keep my eyes closed forever.

Pleased and proud of himself, he put the bag on the kitchen chair, reached inside, and whipped out six brand new arrows. Not long before, he had shown me how to use my bow. The brightly colored feathers flashed through the air and took me by surprise. I fingered one, admiring the newness of the soft, shiny wood, the delicate weight, and the sharp, pointed tip. It was a thoughtful gift and it hit the target.

"Thanks. These are really nice."

"I knew you'd like them."

Subject: Ted
From: Jim Clark

Sat. 12/24: Ted went to Dartmouth for 6:45 and was able to receive his chemo. They were able to insert the IV in on 2nd try with no problem. They left Dartmouth at 9:00 and home by 10:00. I spoke with Brenda, and Ted was resting and a little nauseous. Cat Scan results came back and no new signs of cancer and old areas were reduced. White cell and platelets showed improvement as well.

Merry X-mas
Jim

Christmas at the white, Protestant Clark home on The Plains was filled with tradition. It was against the rules for anyone, even the youngest, to go into the living room until everyone was up. The living room door was shut the night before. This meant the younger ones, namely Jimmy and Dolly, would have to make sure Teddy was out of bed before they could see what Santa had brought. Santa brought one big gift for each child that was left unwrapped on the living room carpet.

Dolly was dressed in yellow Doctor Dentons. Her mop of tight, blond curls covered her small head and one spring-like curl marked the center of her forehead. I liked to pull it down, then watch it spring back into shape. She climbed on Teddy's twin-sized bed and jumped up and down, "It's Christmas. You have to get up! You have to get up!"

Teddy pulled the covers closely around his neck, and mumbled under his breath, "Yeah. I will. Just leave me alone."

Dolly fled from Teddy's room and ran up the back hall stairs to arouse Muffy and me, while Jimmy struggled with Becky and Debbie. By now, Mom and Dad were already up and Mom was making coffee. It wasn't too early—maybe around 7:00 AM.

I heard the scruff scruff of Doctor Denton padding as Dolly made her way around the banister, down the wooden floor hallway, and approached our door. I was peeking out from under the covers, when her three-year-old face bursting with Christmas cheer yelled, "It's time to get up. It's time to get up," and then she disappeared. As much as I wanted to get out of bed, the comfort of the four layers of blankets made it hard to move. I was perfectly cocooned in the sag in the middle of my lumpy mattress. The thought of putting my bare feet on the cold, pine boards and watching my breath escape from my mouth made it even harder. Sometimes, when it got really cold I wore socks to bed. But, this was Christmas, and Dolly and Jimmy were excited to get to the living room. It wouldn't be fair to make them wait very long. I calculated where my bathrobe was and where my slippers were, threw off my covers, and made a mad dash. I had to do it quickly or not at all. As warm air escaped from under the covers and collided with its frigid counterpart, I wrapped myself tightly in a dingy, pale yellow terrycloth robe and slipped into fuzzy, blue slippers.

"Come on, Muffy, you have to get up. Dolly and Jimmy are waiting." I bounced her gently in her bed, as I headed downstairs. Like Teddy, she mumbled under her breath, "I'm comin'."

Entering the kitchen, I spied the Swedish tea ring, made special the day before. The traditional tea ring—baked to perfection, wrapped in cinnamon and sugar, covered with confectionary icing, and sprinkled with cherries and walnuts—was my favorite part about Christmas morning. There it was on the Formica countertop covered in wax paper tempting me. I went to cut a piece, but Mom was there to catch me, "Not until after you have your orange." Another tradition: we had to eat the orange left in the bottom of our stocking before we could eat anything else.

Dad was into counting. He counted how many children he had. He counted how many people attended church on Sunday mornings. He counted how many baskets Ted and I scored. He counted how many eggs his chickens laid. As one sleepy-eyed, tussled-hair child after another staggered into the kitchen, Dad glanced around his kitchen and started to count. He pointed to Mom, then Becky, then Debbie, then Muffy, then me, then Jimmy, and then Dolly. One, two, three, four, five, six, seven. He stopped and asked, "Who's missin'?" Jimmy and I quickly answered, "Teddy."

"Well, go get him up." Dad gave us his full permission.

I grabbed Dolly by the hand and whispered in her ear, "Let's go tickle Teddy."

She scooted off in front of me. Jimmy and I followed. When Teddy heard us outside his door, he pulled his covers over his head and braced himself for the attack. Dolly, Jimmy, and I pounced on him, tugging at the heavy, Indian print blanket. I pulled away one corner of the brown silk binding and exposed his skin. Jimmy and Dolly burrowed in. Twenty tiny digits wriggled across Teddy's neck and made him start kicking—he was roaring when he threw the three of us off. We landed in a heap on one side of his bed. "I'm up," he announced, as he left us in a pile on the floor.

Ted awoke Christmas morning feeling tired, but relieved. He was thinking that he probably could use some more platelets, but that would have to wait until the next day. He was alive. He was home. Perhaps the New Year ahead would bring him better days.

MGH

Adrienne—a name synonymous with Rocky—is a powerful name; and it came with a powerful person with a powerful job. She was a Bone Marrow Coordinator at Massachusetts General Hospital (MGH). After weeks of emailing and talking with her over the phone, the day had arrived for me to meet her in person, January 13, 2004. In order to be the stem cell donor for Ted, I had to be thoroughly examined. Now that the doctors had decided that my blood—even though a mismatch—was good enough to use, they had to see if the rest of me met the health standards. "Health standards." This is something I studied a lot about in my health management and policy courses at the University of New Hampshire. What is medically effective? Is one medical procedure more efficient than another? Who determines what is equitable? What are the standards of practice? I was about to meet all of these head on.

Ted and I were instructed to meet Adrienne in the lobby of MGH at 9:45 AM to begin a busy schedule of testing. We had to call her from bumper-to-bumper traffic on Route 495 to let her know we would be running late.

"I'm sorry, Adrienne. It looks like we'll be late. I'm not sure how long we'll be stuck in this traffic."

"That's okay. Just page me when you get here."

By now, after numerous telephone calls, I was familiar with the soft voice that always conveyed just the right amount of caring. She ended conversations with, "If you have any more questions, don't hesitate to call." I knew by the tone in her voice that she meant it. Having been on the other end of trying to give hope, I was well aware of the delicacy of her position. Yes, she could be trained to do her job, but no amount of in-services could teach her to be herself. Her personality was what this job required. Adrienne's voice was eager to please, eager to reassure, not overly confident, and ready to seek an answer for that which was unknown. She was someone I'd like to sit down with and have a cup of coffee. The ability to make someone feel comfortable in a very uncomfortable situation can't be taught. It is an innate and valuable skill. Adrienne possessed that talent. For me, she was the perfect person in the perfect place, at the perfect time. If there is such a thing as fate, fate had it that we should meet under these circumstances.

Fighting through week-day morning Boston traffic, exiting Storrow Drive and heading toward MGH, is like fighting cancer. If you see the slightest opportunity to squeeze by, you take it. You don't know what the chances are of making it, but you hope the odds are in your favor. You don't look back to wonder if you "should have" because by then it would be too late. Some tractor trailer truck is always going to pull in front of you and block the sign you've been waiting for. You have to seize the moment.

Brenda, eyes doing a last minute peripheral check, punched the gas and merged her way to the stop sign just under the bridge before Commonwealth Ave. Sitting in the back seat, I glanced at my schedule one more time and figured we'd be about twenty minutes late. Ted had been asleep most of the ride down, but was awake in time to observe a homeless man, "There's that guy again. He's been there every time Brenda and I have been in."

I crossed my fingers that it wouldn't take forever for the light to change, but it did. I began to squirm in my seat because there was nowhere to hide. I knew the homeless man might approach our car to ask for money. I took a good long look at what was around me. I checked to see if the car door was locked. To my right, just a foot away from my elbow, was a Pepsi delivery truck, towering over the sea of shorter vehicles. I thought it was going to kiss the side of our car. In back, was a black SUV carrying a commuter talking on her cell phone. In front, was a police officer enforcing the "unknown rules" of this multiple direction intersection as novice drivers attempted to stick the noses of their cars in other drivers' lanes. In the distance, pedestrians bustled among moving cars and dodged cement barricades. Gusts of wind blew pieces of paper as added distraction. Faces were nondescript. I heard a siren in the distance.

To my left was the backdrop of MGH, brick upon brick, looming above the honking horns. The chaos was palpable. Nervously, I ran my tongue over my upper lip. I scratched the inside of my ear. Trucks, cars, and vans moving north, south, east, and west all converged near the same concrete point—near the overpass. A man of medium height was standing in the middle of this intersection. He was an island unto himself. His scraggly salt and pepper beard was about a month old. His matted gray streaked hair hadn't been combed in days. With layers of clothing, he probably weighed about one hundred and forty-five pounds. An out-dated army jacket covered his torso. He shuffled a few steps at a time, first in one direction and then the other. The tips of his fingers poked out from the open ended black gloves as he gripped his heavy sign. "Viet Nam Vet" was scrawled across the rough surface in black paint. As each driver approached, he looked in the glass and reached out a hand. The light changed and Brenda inched forward before he got to us.

She drove safely through the intersection and nudged her way into the left lane, anticipating the left hand turn into MGH. Although I had been to Boston numerous times, it was usually for a concert, museum or sporting event. This was my first visit ever to this renowned hospital and I was taking everything in: doctors dressed in white lab coats; patients being pushed in wheelchairs; and visitors roaming the sidewalks. It was a maze of a human kind. Cars lined up to get into the parking garage closest to the hospital entrance. Fortunately for us, the "Parking Lot Full" sign had yet to block the entryway. Black tar under rubber tires and gray cement on both sides followed us down the narrow hill, around the tight corner, and up beyond the first level. We were lucky to find a space on the fourth level that was just big enough to get the car doors open.

Adrienne warned us that it was going to be a long day. Brenda packed a lunch and her running clothes. I brought my lunch and a new cooking magazine. Ted carried his usual stash of drugs, a bottle of water, and some reading material in a bag. The bag was as pathetic-looking as he—a rumpled, loose bag with no label, no glamour, and no glitz—*not even a pocket handkerchief.* Again, as Bilbo Baggins would say, *how could one survive?* When I glanced at his bag, my first thought was, we can find him something better than that. But then, I second-guessed myself, thinking he was probably content to keep his system intact. It seemed to be working for him. He packed it himself and knew where everything was. I avoided the temptation to find him a nicer bag. The limp bag bumped with every step, against Ted's limp body as he showed me the way to the elevator.

A yellow taxi cab pulled in front of us as we headed toward the sidewalk. One of the hospital attendants was there with a wheelchair, as a heavy-set woman struggled to get out of the back seat. I watched as

Ted slowly and methodically lifted his foot up and over the curb, wobbling his way forward.

"Did you need some help, Ted?" I tried to be nonchalant.

"No. I'll be all right; I'll need to use the bathroom when we get inside. You can page Adrienne."

Knowing Ted and I were safely in the building, Brenda left to do some errands. I approached the high, front desk in the lobby and was greeted by a knowledgeable concierge.

"Could you page Adrienne Harrison, I have her number here." I handed the black uniformed man a piece of paper and glanced down the hallways, all ending up in the lobby. There was a swarm of movement buzzing around me. "Busy bees" moved with intentional precision. The ones in uniforms walked briskly. Fretting patients took their time. In every direction, there were bodies moving—anxiously trying to get somewhere. It was moments before Adrienne arrived.

Her lab coat swayed and her hair bounced up and down as she hurried toward me, "You must be Lucinda, Ted's sister." She had a round face with flushed cheeks. Her eyes were vibrant blue. She radiated life's energy. It was evident that by 10:15 in the morning she had already put in a full day's work.

"Yes I am."

"How's he doing?"

"He's doin' okay. He should be right along; he needed to use the bathroom."

"He's such a great guy."

"I know."

"You know you'll be separated while you give blood. Ted needs a real specialist to handle his veins."

"I know."

"I know he's had some real trouble with that. I hope it goes well today."

"Me too."

"How about you? Ted said you weren't too crazy about giving blood either."

"I'm gonna do my best. I guess if Ted can put up with what he's had to put up with over the last year, I can stand a few pricks here and there."

"I'm sure you'll be fine. We have some great techs."

As Ted approached, Adrienne blurted out, "Hey, Ted, it's nice to see you." Then she dropped her head, "I know it's not nice to have to see me, but you look good." He didn't, but it sounded good to hear.

"Thanks, Adrienne." He smiled as he drew out her long name, emphasizing the A. "I'm going to Bigelow for my pulmonary function test, right?"

"No. We had to change that. You'll do that at the end. I will take your sister now to Cox One so she can get started with her physical. Then, you'll have your blood drawn in Cox Two, while she has more tests in Wang Two. I figure you'll be able to meet up around 12:30 or so for lunch and then we'll let Dr. Wriley know when you're ready to meet with her in one of the conference rooms. Sound good?"

"Sounds like a plan, Adrienne."

Adrienne, who was shorter than both Ted and me, took the lead a few paces in front of us, while I walked side-by-side with Ted. He was unusually quiet. I wanted to know what he was thinking.

Softly I asked, "Are you okay?"

He kept walking as he turned his head toward me, "I don't know if I can do this again."

"Is it the isolation thing?"

"Yeah." His chin began to tremble, "It's gonna be at least five weeks."

"I know. That sure is a long time. I'm so sorry."

We walked in silence the rest of the way down the long hall until our paths split. He went off to the right, and I followed Adrienne to the elevators on the left.

As she pushed the elevator button, Adrienne asked once more, "How's he doing?"

"It's the isolation thing that seems to be bothering him the most. The thought of being cooped up again all that time is really difficult for him."

"There are some pretty decent rooms up on the fourteenth floor. Maybe we'll be able to get him one with a good view." She was being optimistic.

"I sure hope so."

I got confused as Adrienne led me down the patient-filled hallways of the hospital, turning at just the right intersection without hesitation. I could see why I needed the escort. I could barely keep track of what floor I was on, never mind what side of the building. I was impressed that it was part of her job to show me where to go.

Timing is everything, and in true relay fashion, Adrienne handed me off to Tammy, my appointed physician's assistant. "I'll keep in touch with Tammy and when you're all done here, I'll be back to get you." Adrienne's lab coat swished the door jam on her way to run her next lap with her next donor. It was a successful pass. Tammy took over from there. She brushed away a strand of her straight, brunette hair, and looked at me with deep brown eyes.

"Hi, Lucinda. It's nice to meet you. Do you have any questions for me before we begin?" She was friendly, but reserved.

"Not that I can think of right now. But, I'll probably have a million as soon as you are done and out the door."

She smiled before becoming somber. Tammy was entrusted with conveying as much information as possible about the clinical trial being proposed for Ted. She was a true professional and took her responsibility seriously. As stated in the consent form, "A clinical research trial is a study of a treatment, procedure, or medication done in a medical setting, and only includes people who choose to participate." It struck me odd that her first statement was, "You know you do not have to participate in this procedure." It never crossed my mind not to. "I know," I assured. After that was established, she began to explain.

"You will be part of an experimental process of using mismatched blood for a stem cell transplant. They have discovered that sometimes it actually might be better to use mismatched blood than perfectly matched blood but this is still the subject of research, which is why this is a clinical trial. Also, they would rather use donor-related blood whenever possible. When they use a donor who lives in another part of the country, it can become difficult—especially if they need access to more blood. Are you close to your brother?"

"Do you mean close…as in 'do I live near him'?"

A look of acknowledgement flashed across her face as she responded, "I guess I mean both."

"Yes. We are very close. And, yes I live about an hour away from him."

"That's good." She then went on to clarify, "Actually, I don't know anything about your brother and I'm not supposed to. I am here for you. If you have any concerns or questions…that's what I am here for. I will give you my card so you can call me any time. Are you ready for the physical?"

"Sure."

As she took my pulse, blood pressure, and temperature she went through the protocol of medical questions.

"Are you allergic to any medications?"

"Sulpha."

"Are you on any medications now?"

"No."

"Do you have any neurological issues?"

"I do suffer from migraines."

"Just be aware that prior to the collection process you won't be able to take any Aspirin." She made a note in my chart.

As she examined my legs and ankles she noted my varicose veins. "For five days before the blood collection you will be taking shots of Neupogen. Neupogen is used to stimulate production of white blood cells by your bone marrow. Because of this, you may experience pain in your bones and perhaps increased pain with those veins. We will give you a prescription for pain medication in case you need it."

"That's good to know."

"I'm not sure how you'll be taking your shots."

"I have a sister who's a nurse and I was plannin' on havin' her give me the shots."

"That's fine. But, we do like you to have the first injection in a medical setting in case there is a reaction."

"I'm sure my doctor's office would agree to give me the first shot. I've already talked to them about what I'm doing."

"That would work. We'd hate to make you drive down here just for that one shot. By the way, how was your drive in today?"

"Not too bad, but we did get stuck for awhile on 495, and then it was slow on Storrow Drive."

"I try to avoid that."

"Yeah. No kiddin'."

During my physical, Tammy made me feel like a person—not just another guinea pig in another clinical trial. She was efficient and thorough, but at the same time, she took time to relate to me. Although her day was filled with multitasking, like everybody else in the working world, she made me feel important. That was invaluable. There is no way to compute the cost versus the benefit of this kind of quality. Our health care system is filled with inefficiencies and high costs, but when it comes to being cared for, not just "treated," that's the measurement that means the most to me. When Tammy was wrapping things up she asked again, "Do you have any more questions?"

"What has happened to other patients in this clinical trial?"

She lowered her voice and looked toward the wall, "Well, one man has died." And she was quick to add, "But, he smoked, and he had high blood pressure, and he didn't follow any of the doctors' advice."

I thought about that man, trying to visualize what he looked like, as Tammy left the room to page Adrienne. The image of a person being there one day and gone the next came to mind. What did he look like when he died? Working in a long-term care facility I had seen many older persons die. Because they are supposed to die, does that make it any different? The way we leave this earth can be as different as the way we enter it.

"Betty Boop" was on the bathroom floor—long legs sprawled across the linoleum of her assisted-living room when her heart stopped. Merely a few hours before, the head nurse and I were in her room singing: "We love you, Betty, oh yes we do. We don't love anyone as much as you. When you're not with us we're blue. Oh, Betty, we love you." "Geranium Polly" was wearing one of her favorite flowered dresses, waiting to go to Bingo, when she simply slipped away in her over-stuffed Victorian chair next to her gorgeous, pink geraniums. "Elegant Edith," a real lady in every sense of the word, lingered between white cotton sheets for weeks, hooked to oxygen, before her body let her go. Constant visits from hospice kept her pain free and comfortable. I witnessed all of their deaths, and others, too. Of course I wanted to do anything within my power to help my brother live; yet, if he was meant to die, I didn't want it to go badly. It was still too early to tell if he would go, or which way he would go.

Tammy interrupted my thoughts when she poked her head in and introduced me to Dr. McKnight. He was tall and he was thin but he wasn't real thin. He was another friendly, sincere face, and one of the four oncologists on Ted's team. We spoke just briefly. Soon after, Adrienne scooped me up and whisked me off for my next appointments. Adrienne led me down another long hallway. I sang under my breath, like the foursome in *The Wizard of Oz* afraid to enter the forest, "Blood work, chest X-ray, EKG, Oh, my. Blood work, chest X-ray, EKG, Oh, my. Blood work, chest X-ray, EKG, Oh, my." I lost sight of where we were going. I wondered if the great and powerful Oz was behind one of the white, drawn curtains.

At one point I said to Adrienne, "You could use roller skates around here."

She laughed, "Yeah, except I'm not very good on those."

"Really. I've always thought they'd be a lot of fun. I'm going to try them sometime."

"You go right ahead. Sounds like something your brother would like."

"I don't know. We've never talked about it."

Adrienne opened the door to the largest waiting room I'd ever seen. Chairs and sick people spanned the distance of a large banquet hall. For a room this size, with this many people, it was remarkably quiet. I found a comfortable, leather chair and got ready to have my lunch. Adrienne kept me posted, "I'm going to check on Ted. They should be calling you pretty soon." Brenda, returning from her errands, caught up with me in the waiting room.

"How'd your physical go?"

"Fine. I sure am glad that I'm a relatively healthy person. I can't imagine what it would be like if they found some reason they couldn't use my blood. That would be devastating. Are you gonna go runnin'?"

"Yeah. After I check back on Ted, I think I'll go for a quick one. It's still going to be awhile before we meet with Dr. Wriley."

"You might as well. It beats hanging around here. Lord knows you've had your share of waiting around waiting rooms."

"The runnin' has helped me."

"I bet it has. It's good that you are able to do that. Are you plannin' on doin' any races this spring? My racin' days have been over for a long time."

"I might. Are you nervous about having your blood drawn?"

"I'm tryin' to be a big girl about it."

"Ted was gettin' nervous this morning. They've been havin' a lot of trouble gettin' a good vein for him. I hope they have someone good."

"I don't know how I'd be, if they had to poke me like that. I feel so bad for him."

Brenda ate her granola bar while I munched on a peanut butter and jelly sandwich, until my name was called. I gathered up my canvas bag, "See you later."

"Good luck."

On this leg of the relay, I was passed off to "Jamaica Man." Given the number of needles he handled on a daily basis I figured I was in good hands. I was conscious of a long line of chairs, curtains, and lab techs and wondered how many patients filtered through there every hour. As he read my lab slip and started collecting his supplies he sounded surprised.

"Man, they sure do want a lot of blood out of you, lady." His back was to me and he was busy counting his tubes.

"I know, but you don't have to tell me how many tubes they want."

"Oh. Are you a little nervous?"

"Not really. But I do best if I don't look at everything." I was trying to look anywhere but where the needles were.

"No problem, man."

"I also do best if you talk to me." It sounded funny to my ears to say that, but I figured I might as well be upfront with him. After all, he was going to stick me with a needle and hang around me for the next twenty minutes or so.

He looked over my arms, "Is one vein better than the other?"

"No. I think they're both pretty good."

He looked closer and tapped the crook of my right arm, "Yeah. This one looks real good. We'll take this one. Where do you live?"

"I live in East Kingston, New Hampshire. Where do you live?"

"Jamaica Plains."

"Have you been there long?" His accent was pretty strong and I wondered how long he had been in the States.

"Oh. Several years now."

"Do you like it here?" I've always been curious about why people come to the United States, what they like about it, what they don't like about it, and what makes them stay.

"I make a decent livin'."

Liking and making a decent living—were they the same? Jamaica Man made sure my blood was flowing properly and turned to check his paperwork.

"Keep squeezing the ball every few minutes, but not too hard."

I gathered that he didn't want to talk much more and left him alone. Anyway, the tough part was over. I could close my eyes while each tube filled to capacity.

"You're doin' good. How do you feel?"

"I'm fine." But, I could feel the weight of the needle and hoped it would be over soon. The sensation more than the pain was what bothered me.

"So. This blood is for a stem cell transplant?"

"Yeah. It's for my brother."

"Oh. I hope he's treated you well."

"We've had our moments. But, he's been a good brother."

"You're good to do this for him."

"He'd do it for me."

Jamaica Man capped off one tube and started another, "One more to go and you're outta here."

"Thanks. As my brother would say, 'it's been real and it's been good…but it hasn't been real good'."

He chuckled, without comment, as he loaded up the tray of red tubes and marked each one with a black sharpie. When the last glass tube was filled, he took away the needle, gently placed a pad of cotton gauze and secured it with medical tape. He looked at my face and saw that I wasn't looking well.

"Why don't you sit here for a few minutes before you get up."

He didn't have to tell me twice. I watched him retrieve his next patient and waited until some blood returned to my face. By then, Adrienne was back and ready to take me for my chest X-ray and EKG. On our way to Wang Two, she filled me in on Ted.

"The first tech had trouble and they had to call in another one. When I left they were still trying to get his vein."

"Oh great. Just what he needs."

"He's hanging in there though."

"That has to be so tough on him. I wish he didn't have to go through that."

"I know."

The outpatient testing lab waiting area in Wang Two wasn't as large as the previous one, but it was just as busy. Sick people were everywhere. The receptionist took my MGH blue card and told me to take a seat. Brenda had finished her run and joined me in the corner near a brass floor lamp and stack of old *Sports Illustrated* magazines. The aisle between the chairs was narrow. Our knees practically touched those of other waiting patients. I shifted my knees to one side to allow a tall, middle-aged man with his wife to walk by.

"How was your run?"

"Good. It's gettin' a little cloudy out there, but at least there's no snow."

"Are you gonna be able to stay for supper tonight?"

"I think so, if we don't get back too late. I told Kevin not to expect us home. He'll have plenty of homework to keep him busy."

"How's he doin'?"

"Pretty good. I wish he would get involved in more acting."

"I know. He did such a good job with that last play he was in. I made crab chowdah. Do you guys like that?"

"Yeah. That sounds good. Ted will like that."

The receptionist tried to pronounce my name, "Lucinda Mar…"

I saved her the trouble and stood up on Lucinda, "It's Marcoo."

While I was having my chest X-ray and EKG, a skilled technician finally managed to draw Ted's blood. It was a long walk from Cox Two to Wang Two and getting the blood had been tortuous. He was wheeled down to join me in outpatient testing. Ted would also need a chest X-ray and an EKG. We connected in the hall between examining rooms.

"How's it goin', CC?"

I was glad to see him, but could tell by the look on his face that he was hurting. "Just great, Ted. How you doin'?"

"Could be better. Could be worse."

"I know. I heard they had more trouble finding a vein."

"It took them five tries."

"Sorry, Ted."

He shrugged, "What are you gonna do?"

Because we were late getting started, Ted's pulmonary function test had to be rescheduled. It was scheduled after the blood work, the chest X-ray, and the EKG. It was the last test before we could meet with Dr. Wriley. As the three of us waited for Ted to be called, I tried to fill in the gaps. I don't like "gaposis" in conversation.

"Exactly how do they do this test?" I wanted to be able to picture how the pulmonary function test was done.

"They take a tube and you have to blow into it." Ted took on the role of instructor as he filled me in on the details. Shortly into the description, his name was called. Brenda and I remained quiet, as he was wheeled away. With one eye on my magazine and the other on other waiting patients, I thought of Ted. I pictured him behind the closed doors trying to blow as much air into a tube as he possibly could. He would try to prove that he had enough lung capacity to endure the next stem cell transplant.

Adrienne arrived just as Ted was wheeled back into the waiting room. She was ready to go over the rest of the day's agenda.

"We scheduled the conference room for 2:30. Dr. Wriley will be ready to meet with you. I'll bring you down there. Have you had anything to eat?"

"Brenda and I have." I looked at Ted, "Have you eaten yet?"

"No. But I'm not hungry."

"All right." Adrienne looked at her watch, "It's almost 2:00 now, so you won't have to wait too long. Did you want to wait in the conference room?"

We all agreed that would be fine.

I don't remember Adrienne leaving us that day. She had the art of being unobtrusive. Ted, Brenda, and I were quiet while we waited for Dr. Wriley. All other MGH patients, visitors, doctors, nurses, lab tech's, kitchen help, dietary workers, etc., etc. were left behind the closed door. This meeting was confidential. Now, it was time to talk about the next step—one test at a time, one step at a time. Brenda had told me she could only concentrate on one *thing* at a time—the *thing* most pressing. And, this day completed one more *thing*.

The ten-foot long conference room table seemed to go on forever, starting at the door, spanning the room, and reaching for the other side. The four of us didn't need such a large table. Yet, a conference table sets the stage for business and this was a form of business, the business of going about how to save a life.

It was impossible for me to comprehend how Ted was feeling. What would I be feeling if I was in his shoes? Respectfully, I sat on one side of the table with plenty of elbow room. Ted and Brenda sat across from me, with ample space between them. When Dr. Wriley arrived, she took her place at the head of the table. Her petite frame and short black hair belied the strength of her presence, as she took control of the meeting. It was obvious she would take care of business. Her manner was both compassionate and professional. I thought about the dozens of other patients under her care, knowing that Ted was only one of many. How many more meetings had she had on this day?

She reached to shake my hand, "Hi, Lucinda, nice to meet you. I'm Dr. Wriley. I've already met Ted and Brenda. Good to see you both again." And looking directly at Ted she asked, "How are you doing, Ted?"

After months of chemo, the effects of cancer, the day of testing, plus the pressure of the upcoming decision to move forward with another stem cell transplant, Ted looked beaten. It wasn't that someone had taken a bat and covered him in black and blue bruises, but something had scarred him. Like the evening in the Gazebo, his eyes were filled with fear. His chin shook when he answered, "I'm okay." And, he was looking at her for help.

Dr. Wriley took a deep breath and began to explain in detail about the allogeneic stem cell process, something that Ted and Brenda had heard quite a bit about by now. They also had done their research. When Dr. Wriley started talking, I tried to concentrate, but my mind was only able to pick out bits and pieces. It sounded like this: "Yadda, yadda, yadda. There is a twenty percent chance that this will work. Yadda, yadda, yadda. There is a high chance that Ted will contract another form of cancer. Yadda, yadda, yadda. We will be watching closely for graft versus host symptoms, which is likely to occur." Only the most profound combination of words seemed to register. In particular, the "twenty percent chance" figure was what stuck in my mind. What would that mean for Ted? Where would he fall in the percentages? It didn't sound promising to me. Dr. Wriley didn't convince me otherwise, as she handled our consent forms and passed them to each of us. She wanted to be encouraging, "We can hope for the best. Please take as much time as you need to look these over. You don't have to sign them today."

Between my index finger and my thumb, I held this stapled document. It was eleven pages. The "Research Consent Form" outlined all the details of the study beginning with: "Protocol Title: Non-Meyloablative HLA-Mismatched Ex-vivo T-Cell Depleted Stem Cell Transplantation for Hematologic Malignancies," and ending with "Documentation of Consent." There really was no need for me to read any of it; I already knew I was going to sign it, no matter what it said. But, I felt the obligation to make an attempt at understanding the process. In the same way I "half-listened" to Dr. Wriley, I "half-read" the document. I picked out bits and pieces. I took note of specific lines. In particular, this sentence stood out, "It is important for you to know that if you decline to donate after the intended recipient has begun treatments in preparation for transplant, the recipient most likely will die." The "recipient" was Ted. The translation was, unless I signed the document, Ted most likely will die.

The gravity of the situation hit me. This really is life or death. Ted would need to make a decision. If he refused this treatment being offered he might die. If he took his chances and accepted this treatment he might die. Either way, the outcome may not be favorable. Should he resign himself that enough was enough and stay put, or should he take the unproven course? Dr. Wriley asked him the question.

"Ted, what do you want to do?"

He answered with, "I've come this far. What other choice do I have?"

I was thinking, but could not bring myself to say, you don't have to do this. Audible to me, but not to anyone else, was *The Hobbit* chant, *to measure the meaning can make you delay, it's time you stop thinking and wasting the day.* The thought of more tests, more poking and prodding, more chemo, more days in the hospitals, more disabling side effects, and no assurances was more than I could bear. I was thinking, if I were in your shoes, I would just say no. But, I wasn't Ted.

The Show on the Road

After the decision was made, and the tests had been taken, Ted and I were ready for the stem cell transplant to take place, but we had to get by another road-block. The obstacle this time was obtaining permission to use a drug called Medi-507. Ted's team of doctors reviewed existing data on drugs being used to treat side effects of graft versus host symptoms. It was their opinion that Medi-507 would be the most effective. However, it was an experimental drug. The Food and Drug Administration (FDA) had pulled it from circulation as part of the required clinical trial process. Unfortunately, this was when Ted needed it the most. Because of the uncertainty about the availability of the drug, he was, like Beetlejuice, becoming "a little anxious."

Subject: Re: Ted Clark cancer treatment
From: Ted Clark
Date: Mon, 2 Feb 2004
To: Harrison, Adrienne

Hi Adrienne

I have my last chemo tomorrow and I am very anxious to know what the status is about FDA's approval of the medi-507. Although I think the chemo helps to keep the cancer at bay, I'm again starting to get the familiar night sweats and fevers. My sister and I are ready to get the show on the road at Mass General.

Adrienne, like the doctors, had no control over when the FDA would release Medi-507. She could only convey Ted's concern to her superiors.

"*Hi, Ted, I'm sorry to hear that you're not feeling very well. I personally have not heard any news regarding the Medi-507 but I have forwarded your e-mail to Dr. Wriley so that she can respond. I hope that we can 'get the show on the road' ASAP too. We want you to get better soon!"*

As one week flipped to the next, Ted's condition continued to decline. He was growing weaker by the day. Because it was taking so long to get the medication approved, Ted and I would need to be retested. There was more emailing, more phone calls, and more concern.

*From: Ted Clark
Sent: Monday, February 09, 2004
To: Pat & Lucinda; Harrison, Adrienne
Subject: Blood Work*

Hi Adrienne

Lucinda & I plan on going to Mass General on Thursday afternoon (February 12) to redo necessary blood work for my cancer treatment. Is there anything else we have to do?

Ted Clark

*From: Harrison, Adrienne
To: Ted Clark
Sent: Monday, February 09, 2004
Subject: Re: Blood Work*

Hi Ted

We just need to do blood work at this point. You shouldn't be here very long. I will need to meet you so that I can deliver the research samples to our lab right after they're drawn. Sorry to make you guys trudge down here just for blood work. Please be sure to eat and drink plenty of fluids beforehand (I'm sure I don't need to tell you that!). Please have me paged when you arrive. Thanks Ted.

Adrienne

Days later Adrienne sent another message.

Hi Ted

It's just your friendly pain in the butt coordinator at MGH. I didn't want to disturb you with a phone call in case you were resting today but I was hoping that you had a chance to visit your dentist and if so ask if they could fax us a short note detailing your current condition. They can fax it to the number listed below. Thanks Ted. Sorry to be such a pest!

Sincerely,
Adrienne Harrison, Bone Marrow Transplant Coordinator

Every time I spoke with Ted I could feel him slipping away. His voice was not as strong, his outlook was not as great, and his fear that the end was near was taking root. Two years of trying to be upbeat, trying to beat the odds, trying to stay positive was met with adversity. In desperation, even though I knew there was probably nothing she could do, I called Dr. Wriley.

"Do you have any idea when Medi-507 will be released?"

"It looks like it should be any time now. I know Ted has been waiting a long time for it. We're hoping it will be very soon."

Thinking about how shaky Ted's voice was the last time I spoke with him, I couldn't help but say, "I'm afraid it's going to be too late." There was silence on the other end of the phone. I knew Ted was scared, too.

From: Ted Clark
Date: Wed., 25 Feb 2004
FYI Hi Every one

I haven't heard yet that FDA approved the new drug............ waiting is the worst part. I had to go into Concord hospital today for blood transfusion, my blood counts were getting too low. Hopefully next Monday we can get the ball rolling.

Driving from work one day I realized that Ted's fiftieth birthday was coming up—March 9th. Of the seven of us, his was the only birth date that my dad could remember. I couldn't help but think it could be Ted's last. Would he want to celebrate it? What could we do for him to make it a good one? I thought about his favorite birthday meal. Would he be up for Mom's homemade spaghetti sauce? It was worth a try. I called him from my cell phone.

"Hi, Ted. You have a birthday comin' up. Would you want us all to come to your house and bring you a spaghetti dinner?" Knowing he would not be able to come to East Kingston, the only option was to bring the party to him. In the past, it never would have occurred to me to do this, but things had changed. I thought there may be hesitation on his part, but there wasn't. He didn't even pause to think about an answer.

"Sure. That would be good."

Though his answer caught me by surprise, I was pleased he liked my suggestion, "Great. I will give the others a call and hope that everyone can make it. How about this Sunday?"

"We don't have any plans that I know of. I'll check with Brenda, but I think that'll be fine."

"Tell her she doesn't have to do anything. We'll bring everything we'll need."

Even though she didn't "have to do anything," I was conscious of the intrusion into their lives. How invasive was I? How bold? I picked up the phone and invited myself and a whole bunch of people to their home. An onslaught of the Clark Clan involves a lot of people. It couldn't be helped. You marry a Clark, you marry a family. The vow you take is for better or for worse.

I had enough cell phone reception to continue calling as I drove down Route 125. Passing the truck-stop diner, I searched for Jimmy's number. Once again, the troupe, the posse, the cavalry would be rounded up to try to contain this attack on our family. Remarkably, each sibling I spoke with said they could make it Sunday, even though it was on short notice. All they wanted to know was what time and what to bring. Everyone thought it was a good idea. It didn't take much to put the menu together—"Mom, you bring your spaghetti sauce. Becky and Barbara, bring salads. Debbie, bring drinks. Muffy, bring garlic bread. Dolly, bring the cake." What do you put on a 50th birthday cake for someone whose days may be numbered, "Good luck, best wishes, hope you are around for the next one?" I would help Mom with the spaghetti sauce. Knowing we didn't have much time, the plan came together quickly.

When Pat and I arrived, with paper plates and a pot of spaghetti sauce, the house was quiet. Kevin was on the computer, and Ted was in his chair. Brenda greeted us at the door and let us unpack.

"Come on in. I was just straightening up in the kitchen."

I felt the need to apologize, "Sorry about the intrusion. I hope you don't mind us all coming tonight."

"Oh. No problem. We weren't doing anything anyway." Besides, what choice did she have?

I put my bags on the table and walked over to Ted. He was wearing a long sleeve white cotton shirt and a green baseball hat. He smiled as I reached to give him a hug and a kiss on the cheek, "Happy Birthday, Ted."

"Thanks for comin'."

"You don't think we'd let this one get by without bothering you. It's the big 5 0."

"I guess it is."

Ted was wistful. He showed signs of pensive sadness. The invisible ghost that haunted my thoughts, and Ted's cancer, would not go away. It lurked in every crevice of his house, oozing up through the cracks in the floor boards, and slithering down the staircase. It crept up on him when he wasn't looking, and when he was. He rubbed his eyes, he blinked, but it was still there. Was it time to stop running from this ghost and turn to face it head on? How do you embrace a ghost? Ted's longing to know what the future held for him and his unfulfilled desire to have these ghostly sightings disappear were elusive. He knew the ghost was there, but every time he reached out to grab it, it slipped through his hands.

Becky and Ron arrived with their salad and a cooler filled with drinks. Mom and Dad followed them in. Debbie and her husband Wolfgang bumped into Dolly as they reached the granite step at the same time. Jimmy, Barbara and Muffy were the last to knock on the door. Dave and Dolly's husband Scott couldn't make it. Coats and boots were left in the entryway as people trailed from the living room, to the dining room, to the kitchen. Family greetings and newsworthy chatter dribbled from one relative to the next. Side-bar conversations about Ted's condition were held with Brenda out of Ted's hearing. Happy thoughts and sad thoughts bounced up and down like basketballs in a drill.

Ted liked being kept in the game and the more people arrived, the better he began to look. For a brief period, Ted could wrap his troubles into a big, tight ball and shoot them out of sight. He knew that Ron, the high school teacher, had been working with his students on a robot. The annual Robotics Tournament had been held the day before at the Verizon Center in Manchester.

"Hey, Ron. How did the competition go yesterday?"

"Gufaw, guffaw, guffaw," Ron amused himself with thoughts of the day before, "It went pretty well but we didn't make the finals. The kids had a good time, but our robot got pretty beat up."

"What was your problem? Aren't you supposed to be the physics genius?"

"Well – guffaw, guffaw, guffaw – we were at a bit of a disadvantage."

"No excuses now…"

"All the other teams had an engineering firm to sponsor them." He looked toward Pat, who was talking with Muffy, "Maybe next year we can get some help from Pat…"

Ted smiled looking in the same direction, "That might help."

I circulated through the rooms, listening in on various conversations. Dolly was talking to Wolfgang about her recent marathon, "I hit the wall at mile twenty-three." Muffy and Jimmy were rehashing Dave's retirement party, "It was sad, but it turned out to be a real celebration of his twenty years. His ex-players gave him a real tribute." And Becky, as if drawing up a needle, was pulling information out of Brenda, "How much longer will you wait for Medi-507 before trying something else?" In true nursing style, she asked the tough questions. Mom was standing at the stove and had her back to Brenda and Becky. She bit her bottom lip, as she took the lid off the steaming Revere Ware pan, and began to stir the pot. She breathed in the scent.

The smell of oregano and basil drifted from the kitchen. It wafted from the stove, over the dining room table, through the open doorway and into the living room. It tugged at our senses. One huge pot of boiling water made the pasta al dente. Crisp lettuce, red tomatoes, and green peppers flashed colors of spring. On the counter, a white frosted sheet cake with "Happy Birthday Ted" waited. Basking in the aroma of past and present we prepared to break apart the long, white loaf of Italian garlic bread calling our collective names.

When children are about to be born, we bring gifts and shower our guests with food. At weddings, we gather around decorated tables and toast with wine and champagne. Funerals bring us together over demi plates of deli sandwiches, chips, pickles, and chocolate brownies.

Birthday celebrations wouldn't be the same without tasty morsels and meals fit for a king. Equal in all cultures, food is part of our heritage and our tradition.

We siblings, our spouses, our mother and father, and our children each found a seat. Kevin was left standing at the blue kitchen counter. It took two tables, one in the kitchen and one in the dining room to accommodate the lot of us. As the filled to-the-brim bowl of hot spices and cooked hamburger landed in front of Ted, I did not fear that I would be short-changed. Watching him slowly lift the spoon and scoop up some sauce, I could hear my mother's voice, "Teddy, don't take too much. There are more people at this table!"

I jumped over "D Loves P" and the cracks in the cement walk and hurried to the porch. Church was over! Thank God. Pushing Jimmy out of the way and catching up to Teddy, I rushed into the house.

Even if I wasn't hungry, which I was, I couldn't wait to eat. Roast beef, soaking and spitting in its juices was sweet and the smell triggered a visceral response. Nothing tasted better than Mom's roast beef followed by apple pie, except maybe—her spaghetti sauce. And no one appreciated Mom's cooking more than Teddy. For this, Mom was grateful. She loved the fact that Teddy loved her cooking.

I, on the other hand, didn't appreciate this fact. Sitting next to him at meal time was, at the least, suspenseful. I watched as a small plate piled high with First National white bread disappeared one slice at a time and arrived at my right hand nearly demolished. I took a lonely slice and watched as hard butter, like pie crust folding over a rolling pin, ripped a hole up the center. Then, I eyed the heaping white mound of mashed potatoes. In seconds, it was cut in half. It took my breath away. My mother saw it too, "Ted, put some of that back." Reluctantly, he refilled some of the bowl. He couldn't help himself when the roast beef came his way. Again, he took more than he should have. As he reached for the gravy, I dared to stab a thick piece of roast beef from his plate and slap it on my own. I watched him cover his plate in brown, delicious gravy and hollered, "Hey! Save some for me."

There was plenty of Aunt Eleanor's red, Austrian-derived sauce to go around. There was plenty of garlic bread, salad, and pasta too. No one was going to go away from this birthday table hungry. For sure, Ted's appetite had decreased and he took considerably smaller portions. I wished his appetite was like when we were kids. He nibbled at his salad, and had difficulty getting down the carrots. The way he chewed looked like it hurt his teeth. Shaking, he reached for his glass of water—not beer, and not wine. Swallowing and digesting had become an unpredictable process. He was never sure what was going to stay down. Like mixing hamburger, ketchup, and mashed potatoes in a blender—he continued to experiment. Unfortunately, he no longer had an iron stomach.

"Ted," Jimmy asked, "remember when you used to run in those road races with Pat and Dave?"

"Yeah, that was always a trip."

"I never could get how you could eat and then run. That would have bothered the heck out of me."

"It never bothered me."

"I know. You could eat a McDonald's cheeseburger and then run a ten K."

I piped in, "I thought I could beat you that time you ate a heavy meal at my house and I challenged you to run to the end of Sanborn Road. We were in our late twenties or so. I had been runnin' a lot and you hadn't been runnin' at all. It didn't matter, you still beat me."

He looked up from his plate and smiled, "You should have known better."

"I know. I'm a slow learner."

Becky and Debbie were in the kitchen lighting his cake when I heard laughing in the other room.

"I looked over and Teddy's eyes were bugging out. The next thing I knew he was throwing up in his face mask." Brenda was chuckling as she told about the time Ted vomited in his mask when they were scuba diving.

"That is so gross," Jimmy smirked looking right at Ted.

The constant waves bobbing him up and down underwater churned his stomach and made him hurl. It was a good story and one we had all heard before. Ted hadn't lived that one down.

Becky and Debbie carried the cake into the living room. Ted waited patiently at one end of the table.

"Happy Birthday to you. Happy Birthday to you. Happy Birthday, dear Teddy…happy birthday to you."

None of us can sing very well and it's pathetic to hear us under good circumstances. The added dimension of not knowing how many more birthdays Ted would celebrate left our voices fading on the last round. As he bent over to blow out the candles, we knew what he was wishing for. We all wished for the same thing.

Remarkably, on his actual birthday, March 9th, one of his wishes did come true. Ted received the call that the FDA had released Medi-507 and it could be used. Jimmy let us know.

Subject: Update on Ted
From: Jim Clark
Date: Tue, 9 Mar 2004
Update on Ted: Happy 50th Bro.

- *Ted got a nice B-day gift today with the FDA's approval of the Medi-507 drug to help with the effects of Graft vs Host*
- *Ted will go in on Monday 3/15 to Mass General to have Hickman Port put in. I believe Chemo will begin on Monday also. I was all ready to take him in on Wed am, but that all got changed.*
- *Brenda is in Rhode Island and the boys are with Ted*
- *Ted will pretty much hang loose this week and may have blood work in Concord.*

That's all I know. Jim

As Ted had said, "waiting is the worst part." Waiting for Medi-507, and now, waiting to be admitted to MGH was grueling. Each day that he had to wait his blood counts worsened. His shortness of breath increased. His blood pressure was frighteningly low. I spoke with him on Sunday, March 14th and ached from the nearly one-sided conversation. Mandy was coming home from NYC and I had to pick her up at the bus station in Newburyport, MA. I knew she wouldn't want to have to drive another couple of hours to Loudon but it was in the back of my mind. There was a sense of urgency that I couldn't ignore. Waiting in the car for Mandy's bus to pull in, I went back and forth—should we go to see Ted or should we not, should we got to see Ted or should we not, should we go to see Ted or should we not? I let Mandy make the decision.

It was a comfort to see my daughter—the nurse, the child grown into an adult, the friend she had become. I watched her say good-bye to her high school friend and pull her suitcase over to the curb. She looked tired from the long bus ride and, as usual, had her long thick black hair pulled back in a bun. I was conscious of her height as she bent over to give me a hug. We put her bags into the trunk and I let her take the wheel.

"How are you doin', Mom?"

I couldn't hold back my tears. She knew how bad things were getting, "I spoke to Ted earlier and he is so bad. I'm wondering if we should go see him, but I don't want you to have to keep driving all the way to Loudon. I don't know what we could do for him if we did go."

"Mom, is that what you want to do?"

"I think so."

"Then, that's what we'll do."

She took over from here, pulling out of the parking lot and onto Route 95. From Newburyport to Loudon, I filled her in on the news. We were waiting for Ted to be admitted. Then, I could start my Neupogen shots. By the time we got to his driveway, she had the picture. Yet, I don't think she was prepared to see Ted in the condition he was.

Frail, short of breath, and white, he did not move from his chair. I know he was glad to see us, but he was hurting too much to let us know. It was all he could do to say "hello" and it was all I could do to bend down, reach over the arm of the recliner, and whisper in his ear, "I love you." His voice was almost too soft to hear, "I love you, too."

"See who I brought to cheer you up. Another nurse to check up on you."

"Yeah. But, she's a real pretty one." Gasping between his words, he tried to be sociable.

"I know. Don't you think she takes after me?"

"I don't know about that... Maybe when you were a lot younger." It was meant to be funny, but he was too weak to smile.

Mandy stepped closer to his chair and he could barely raise his arms, "Hi, Ted. Do you want me to take your blood pressure?"

"We don't have a blood pressure cuff."

"And, I didn't bring one."

"Guess you're not too efficient, are you?" He was having trouble keeping his eyes open.

"Hey, sometimes I mess up, too."

"When did you get back from New York?" He often asked how Mandy liked living in the big city.

"My mom picked me up in Newburyport a couple of hours ago and we came straight here."

"Gee. You didn't have to do that just for me. Do you want something to eat?"

"No. We're all set. My mom promised me something good when we get home."

"I bet she did. There has to be some reason to come home."

I added, "Isn't that the truth?"

We tried to keep it light, but there was nothing light about it. Brenda was worried and told us they were expecting to admit him to MGH in the morning. I wanted her to call the doctor and tell them he might not make it through the night. I was afraid for both of them. What if he stopped breathing in the middle of the night? What if she couldn't get an ambulance here quick enough? She was self-sufficient, but what was her breaking point?

"Brenda, is there anything you need me to do?"

As usual, she refrained from asking for any help, "Not that I can think of. I've already talked with the doctors. They know his condition."

Mandy and I visited for a short time until Ted fell back asleep. Not wanting to wake him up, we tiptoed toward the door. I turned once more to Brenda, "Please. If you need anything or if anything changes…give me a call." She assured me that she would. As if pulling down a shade, her eyes dropped to the floor, "I will." That night passed without my phone ringing.

The next morning, I awoke to thoughts of Ted. As with any consuming fear—you wake up thinking about the same thing you went to sleep obsessing over. My first thought was, Ted must be alive because we never got a call. The fact was, he was living and he was breathing but he wasn't really alive. (Ted was in critical condition but his heart was strong.) When Brenda arrived at the hospital she required a wheelchair to get him into the Donor Center. Upon examining Ted, the nurses in the Donor Center became alarmed. They were not used to seeing such low blood counts for someone who was about to undergo a stem cell transplant. They needed to consult with his doctors, administer more tests, and start a transfusion before Ted could be brought to his assigned room.

While Brenda struggled to get Teddy admitted, the rest of us struggled in silence. Muffy sent an email that put it into writing.

Subject: Update on Ted
From: Muffy Faucher
Date: Mon. 15 Mar 2004

Hi Family,
I am feeling the need for more communication as to how Teddy is doing. Could we start an e-mail journal or telephone tree of some kind? I had suggested earlier to have each person take a day of the week and find out by calling the hospital or visiting and then getting back to the others. Becky would be in charge of Mondays (including today), Debbie would be Tuesdays, me Wednesdays, Lucinda Thursdays, Jimmy Fridays, Dolly Saturdays, and Mom and Dad Sundays. Does anyone have the numbers of Mass. General and information on when to call or when to visit? Joey might be able to go today but I am not sure. Thanks, Muffy

Given the number of phone calls that would need to be made to keep everyone in the loop, this was an excellent solution. I thought it was a great suggestion and so did everyone else. Why hadn't we started this sooner? It didn't matter, it went into effect immediately. Later that day, she sent another message.

Hi family, This is something what I had envisioned us doing. (This would be Becky's job because it is a Monday): As of 8:15 pm tonight Teddy had not checked into a room yet so we don't have a room number, but he is in the Ellison Building on the 14th floor at Mass. General. The hospital phone number is 617-724-5410. Brenda brought him in and it was expected that he would have the port put in today and start chemo and have blood work done. Lucinda has talked to the coordinator today. Mandy is home this week and Cindy and Mandy (and maybe Mom) are planning to go to Boston tomorrow (Tuesday) to visit. We have appointed Mom the "visiting coordinator" so if you are planning to visit, please inform her first. Thanks, Muffy

It was a relief to know he was in the hospital, and he was safe, for the time being. Tuesday, Pat, Mandy, Mom, and I drove to Boston. He was out having a battery of tests when we got to his room. As hoped for, he had a room with a view. The four of us spread out, looking over his belongings, his bulletin board, his vacant bed, and his bicycle. I looked out the expansive, rectangular windows and saw joggers running along the Charles. A bridge connecting one side of the Charles River with the other was sprinkled with trucks, buses, and cars. Pedestrians looked like miniature moving mannequins in a shadow box. All was quiet on the outside.

A pleasant, professional-looking, short nurse with medium length black hair wheeled my brother into his room. Her name, ironically, was Dorothy. It was ironic in three ways. The youngest and sweetest of our siblings was named Dorothy, even though she goes by Dolly. Ted's name, Theodore, sounded out backwards is Dorothy. And, like Dorothy in the *Wizard of Oz*, Nurse Dorothy was about to befriend a "Cowardly Lion." Together, they would peek behind the curtain to see what the great and powerful Oz would have in store for them. None of us could ever forget her name.

She greeted us with a gracious smile, "Hi, my name is Dorothy. I'm one of Ted's nurses. He can visit for a bit until he has to go for his pulmonary function test. Did you have any questions for me?"

"How's his bilirubin count?" Mom wanted to know.

"It's still pretty high. The doctors don't want to start the new drug and the chemo until that comes down."

"I hope that happens quickly."

"We're working on it." She glanced around the room and added, "Anything else before I go?"

"No. I guess not right now."

Ted had regained some of his sense of humor and he joked with her as she left the room, "Don't hurry back…"

She looked over her shoulder and gave him a wink.

It was no wonder that Ted was acting more like himself. After receiving three blood transfusions the day before, he must have felt human again. Ted was reincarnated—like a vampire supplied with fresh, nourishing red cells. He had come back from the dead.

Pat asked, "Is there anything we can get for you?"

"I could use some Gatorade."

After he was whisked away for his pulmonary function test, we had lunch in the cafeteria and bought him a supply of Gatorade at a local market. When we returned to his room, it was empty. Ted was not back yet. The white blanket and white top sheet were thrown aside. Running shoes were pushed under his bed. A blank menu and a copy of *National Geographic* were on his nightstand. The tall, intrusive I.V. pole was at the head of his bed.

"Do you want to wait for him to come back?" I asked Mandy.

"I do need to get back to the city. If we go now I can probably catch the 2:00 bus."

"Mom, did you want to stay longer?" I wanted to make sure she was okay to go.

"I'm okay, I've seen him now, and will try to get in again later this week. We can go."

"Pat, what do you think?"

"Whatever you want."

"It could be awhile. I'm happy now that I've seen him. We can go."

Leaving the Gatorade on his bed-side table, we felt a new surge of hope. The show was on the road.

Five Million CD Thirty-four Stem Cells

I punched in the code and listened to my voice message. Ted started out on a high note, "Hey, Lucinda. This is Ted. I've been trying to get a hold of ya. It seems like, ummmm, whenever I do I just can't get through. Anyway…ummmm, I'm officially neupogenic, which means I don't have any white cells left." He chuckled, and then his voice began to crack. "So…" His voice dropped lower before he could regain his momentum, "I hope your treating yours are good." What he meant to say was, "I hope your treating cells are good." Resigned, he continued, "Anyway, when you have a chance, give me a call. Thanks. Bye."

How would it be possible that I might be able to breathe new life into my brother? The thought defied comprehension. Like sitting in a cramped seat in an airplane and looking out the window over a vast sea of untouchable clouds, the view seems far from real. If you're not an engineer or perhaps a scientist, you cannot believe your eyes. I could not believe what was in front of me. I was in my office at my desk, hoping that I would not get interrupted, when I returned Ted's call.

"Hi, Ted. I got your message."

"Yeah. I was havin' trouble with your phone, I don't know why."

"I don't either, but at least you did get through."

"Have you heard from Adrienne?"

"No. Now that I know things are moving, I'll give her a call."

"She said she'd call you."

"Well, maybe she's havin' trouble, too. I'll call her."

"That's probably a good idea. Do you know when you start the shots?'

"I was supposed to start them on Friday, but that may have changed. How are you doin'?"

"I'm feelin' okay. How are your super cells?"

"They're just great. Don't worry about not being able to use the remote."

There was a knock on my door and I had to cut him off, "I'll catch yeah later. Get some rest."

Pushing my thoughts of Ted to the back of my brain, and fighting back my tears, I greeted a prospective resident's family member. (By this time I had changed jobs and was working as the Marketing Director at an assisted living community.) He was coughing and noticeably not feeling very well. I didn't want to be rude but I needed to keep my distance. Instead of shaking his hand, I smiled as best I could and offered an explanation.

"I'm so happy you are here, but I really cannot afford to get a cold. I'm sorry if I can't shake your hand." My biggest worry over the past few months was that I would get sick just when it was time for the transplant. T'was the season, and I lived in mortal fear of the flu.

"No problem. I think my mom and dad are ready to sign up."

Fortunately, he was a client with an understanding nature, and I trusted that I had not offended him. We had met on a number of other occasions, and a congenial rapport had been established. He had other things on his mind and seemed to take it in stride. The meeting went well and he signed on the dotted line.

When I stole a few minutes, I connected with Adrienne and she confirmed that I was supposed to start the series of Neupogen shots on Saturday. The series of shots included four days at home, and then the fifth one in Boston—on the first day of harvesting. This presented a minor problem. Originally, I was going to have the first shot in my doctor's office in Exeter where they could monitor me for any adverse reactions. I certainly didn't want to drive to Boston. How could I do this on Saturday? I called Becky that night.

"Beck, they want me to start the shots on Saturday. My doctor's office won't be open."

"Maybe we can do it in the lobby of the emergency room at Exeter Hospital."

"You think that would be okay?"

"Well. We would be right there. And, if you have any reaction I could get you in there pretty fast."

I thought it over for a bit. It sounded kind of odd. I envisioned myself sitting in the lobby, with people all around, and Becky giving me a shot. The alternative was to call MGH and make arrangements to go there. I didn't like the thought of that.

"Do you really think that would be okay?"

"I don't know why not. As long as we can have access to the hospital we should be all right."

I trusted her judgment and agreed that we would go to Exeter Hospital Saturday morning, hoping that I didn't have a reaction.

Climbing into her car, I cleared away nursing debris—stethoscope, plastic cups for urine samples, and a medical supply bag. I saw the square, red plastic container labeled in black ink "Danger. Biohazard Material." "Gee, Beck, if you get stopped by the police they might think you're a drug dealer."

She laughed and threw an *American Journal of Nursing* into the back seat. Being a visiting nurse, she had to carry everything with her. I examined my seat closely before I sat down. I was afraid I might get stabbed in the butt with a needle.

On the drive over, she came up with plan B.

"We can sit in the parking lot in front of the Emergency Room. I can give you the shot in the car."

"You think so?"

"It'll be just as good as goin' inside. We'll be right there."

Though it sounded kind of iffy to me, it had to be done. "Okay. Whatever you say."

With the engine running to keep us warm, Becky dug into her bag. We were in the front seats of her car when she drew up the needle and prepped my lily-white belly with antiseptic. I could only imagine what someone would think if they saw us—me with my shirt pulled up exposing my waist and Becky inserting a needle into it. It didn't really hurt—it was kind of like a bee sting. We waited for any reaction.

"So. Who's taking you in on Wednesday?"

"I think Jim and Mom are gonna go with me."

"Too bad Pat has to be away."

"I know, but with all you guys around, I'll be fine. He knows I'll be in good hands."

"Will they give the stem cells to Ted right away?"

"That's what they said. After they take mine and filter them in the stem cell machine, they bring them right to him and start the transplant."

"How long will it take?"

"They said it can take from five to six hours for them to collect my cells."

"Will they be able to collect what they need in one day?"

"They told me to be prepared to come in for two days and maybe three."

"Are you nervous?'

"Not really. Like Brenda, I'm trying to concentrate on one thing at a time."

"How are you feeling now?"

"So far. So good."

"I think we've waited long enough. I think it's safe enough now to go."

Each day, Sunday, Monday, and Tuesday, Becky continued to give me the shots. As expected, there was some aching in my back and some fatigue. It was nothing that required medication. Ted, experienced in taking Neupogen, had told me to walk. I took his advice and walked every day. Come Wednesday, March 24th, I was ready for my stem cells to be collected.

I awoke at 4:00 AM to incredible throbbing in my jaw. A cracked tooth that had been bothering me for months decided to give me a pain in my mouth—it was not a good way to start the day. Not able to take any Aspirin (that was not allowed before a stem cell collection) I tried to ignore the increasing irritation. Showering, I grew more and more worried. What if they won't let me give my blood today because of a problem with my tooth? All the months of planning, calculating, and preparing had led up to this morning. I managed not to get sick, but now I had a toothache. I didn't think it was an infection—I thought it might be because of the Neupogen. Putting on my make-up (it is better to look good than to feel good) I got ready for Jimmy to pick me up. I walked across the path to Mom's and waited for him to come.

"Hi, Mom. You ready to go?"

"I just need to brush my teeth and I'll be ready." She disappeared into the bathroom and I sat at the kitchen table.

I saw Jim's black Subaru Outback speed up the incline and abruptly turn the corner into Mom's driveway just missing the rock wall. Jim was always in a hurry. He jammed on the brakes and jumped out of the car, hustling to the front door. With a concerned look on his face he greeted me with a hug.

"How you doin'?"

"Just fine, except I have a mega toothache."

"Where did that come from?"

"I don't know, but I wish it would go away. I think it's coming from a cracked tooth that I have. It might be the Neupogen that has aggravated it."

"How's Mom?"

She came around the corner as I was saying, "She's ready to go."

Dad decided it would be too long a day for him. He sauntered out of his bedroom in his cotton, older men's two-piece pajamas. Heavy-handedly, he patted his hair, aware of the white clumps sticking straight up. Child-like, he rubbed his eyes and wiped away his sleepy seeds as he wished us good luck. "What time do you think you'll be back?"

"It's hard to tell. Probably sometime before supper."

In an effort to beat the horrible traffic into Boston, we left at 5:00 AM. Walking to the car I took a moment to stare at my favorite tree—the one that stands alone, across the street, in the middle of an open field. In all the years I have lived on Sanborn Road with houses going up and the world changing around me, this tree has remained steadfast. It has been loyal to me. My children slid down the hill and toppled over in the snow at its base. It watched them brush off the snow and trudge back up the hill. In perfect formation it starts with a solid trunk and then branches out in the shape of an umbrella. Its branches are magnificent—capturing morning's light and embracing night's blackness. Daily, it tempts me to stop and look, and I do. It appears omnipotent and I am respectful of its presence. It is magical. I yearn to have a twig of its mystical power. What does it see as mist crawls up its base and evaporates under its spread? What does it feel as the harsh winds of winter weather its bark, and the sun bakes its limbs? Will it be there forever? I feel reassured knowing that it will be there when I return.

Dad's rooster crowed as we took our seats. It is dark—there are no street lamps on Sanborn Road. Jimmy switches on his headlights as he turns the key. Passing our neighbor's farm, I see flashes of white. Their feisty flock of geese is ducking in and out of the shadows across the cropped remains of corn stalks. I love their wooden sign, dug deep in the corner of the knoll by the road, enticing the adventuresome connoisseur, "Goose Eggs for Sale." This is not a sign I will see on Cambridge Street.

We made good time and arrived at MGH Donor Center around 6:30 AM. I took a seat while I waited for operations to begin. The admitting clerk was still starting up her computer. When she was ready to get her day underway, she asked for my baby blue card. I felt privileged to have this passport in my pocket. I gladly handed it over. As she typed away she asked the required questions. I thought about my aching tooth. Should I say something or not? I decided not to. After she was done taking my blood pressure and making sure I didn't have the flu, or a temperature, I waited to be called to my bed. Mom and Jim had gone to check on Ted and about this time Mom returned (Jim had to go to work.)

"How's your tooth?" Mom asked.

She said it loud enough that one of the Donor Center nurses stopped and looked directly at me.

"What is the matter with your tooth?"

"It's pretty achy. I think it's from being cracked and I think it got aggravated from taking the Neupogen."

She went off to call one of Ted's team doctors, Dr. Miles. She didn't look happy. Mom and I looked at each other and didn't say a word. We just prayed.

I was assigned to Nurse Ginger who began preparing me for the collection. Ginger, a mature woman, was closer in age to me than others I had encountered. She was medium height, medium weight, and had medium brown hair. Yet, there was nothing medium about her. She was extraordinary. One word described her actions—tender. She was relatively new to the Donor Center and still in her probationary period. Her supervisor, like *Black Hawk Down*, would not leave a fallen patient while on her watch. She hovered over Ginger, making sure everything was done correctly. Ginger was thorough, calm, and conscientious about everything she did. They decided to go ahead and get things started while they waited for word from Dr. Miles. Ginger and I would spend the day collecting blood, and getting acquainted.

"Have you gone to the bathroom?"

"Yes, I have."

"Good. You know you won't be able to get up for about six hours after you are hooked up. You will need to ask for a bedpan if you need to go during the day."

"I got that part."

I sat my butt on the edge of the hospital bed and swung both legs over the edge. Thank goodness I didn't have to wear a johnny. With both arms and hands spread out, in prayer-like fashion, I let her examine both arms. The space felt congested, with a chair on one side and a big machine on the other. I kept thinking someone was going to trip. (Sorry, but that might have made me chuckle.) There was another bed and another set-up in the same room, but I was the only one giving on that morning. If needed, curtains could be drawn.

"We need to give you your shots of Neupogen and then draw some blood."

I replied, "Whatever you want to do." I was at their disposal.

She gave me the shot and sent my blood to be tested. They needed to get a STAT white blood count before they could begin collecting. While waiting for the results, Dr. Miles appeared at the foot of my bed. He was about five-feet tall and had beautiful, brown skin.

In a very strong accent his kind demeanor came through, "How are you feeling? I hear you have a problem with your tooth."

"It's throbbing, but I really think it's from a tooth that's been cracked. It's been bothering me for awhile."

He came closer so that he could look in my mouth, which I opened wide for him.

His tiny hands probed the inside of my mouth and I hardly felt a thing. He had the smallest pair of hands on a man that I had ever seen. They came in handy for a doctor. He did not see anything that appeared to be red or swollen.

"I don't think there's an infection. We'll let you give today."

My whole body, from my scalp to my toenails, relaxed. "Thank you!"

I could have cried, but I didn't. Mom, who had been anxiously standing by my bed, felt the same way. Our eyes locked and the look on her face said, "Thank God." I nodded back, "Amen."

Ginger tapped the bulging blue vein of my right arm, swabbed it, and inserted a 17-gauge needle. I wasn't looking but I felt the extra large needle go in. She put a pillow under my elbow and made sure my arm was straight. Gently repositioning it until it looked right to her, she said, "You don't want to move that arm. Let me know if you need anything." Then, she walked around to the other side of my bed and repeated the process with my left arm, but used a smaller 18-gauge needle.

Like Bilbo Baggins on a *Hobbit's Holiday,* my blood began its greatest adventure—*to there and back again.* The 17-gauge needle drew bright red blood out of my body. From there it traveled through a plastic connecting tube and was pumped into a cell separating machine (CSM). I liked to think of CSM as a female because of her function—

nurturing and cradling life-forming cells. She was a dingy shade of white (I would have preferred her to be a soft pink) approximately four-feet tall and two and a half feet wide. CSM was about the size of an old, Italian grandmother. The machine swallowed my blood, flipped it around and around, and regurgitated it in a changed composition. The black base with a black cylinder, in the middle of her belly, spun out the red cells, white cells, and platelets. Only the super cells, as Ted and I referred to them, were allowed to stay.

All unwanted cells returned via the 18-gauge needle and another connecting plastic tube. This is half the journey of the allogeneic, CD thirty-four stem cell transplant. The other half would be when my cells are given to Ted. CD refers to a cluster of differentiation. The number thirty-four designates the order in which each individual stem cell was discovered—thirty-four came after thirty-three. CD thirty-fours are the kick-ass stem cells of the blood underworld, the ones that decide whether cells will become red, white, or platelet. Powerful, they are. CSM prepared my blood to save Ted's life.

A clump of brownish, wavy hair flopped over Ginger's forehead as she checked and rechecked all the tubes, machines, and blood collecting equipment. She kept pushing it aside with her forearm. The pumping would continue for about five hours, and Ginger would remain near my side. She had to monitor my blood pressure, the machine, and me. Another nurse filled in when she went on break, but I was never left unattended. The set-up and breakdown took about an hour. I was prepared for a long day.

Ginger handed me a nerf-like, pink ball with MGH stamped on it, and told me to keep squeezing it gently. (I keep this souvenir hidden in my bureau drawer.) As she bent over to examine the cylinder she explained, "I have to watch the color. The collection needs to be pinkish, not too red and not too white." Hummm, I thought to myself, "Shaken, not stirred."

During my visit for my physical I had a tour of the Donor Center. I did not want to stare. I couldn't remember the details. I wasn't sure, but I didn't think anyone was watching TV. I was pretty sure no one was reading a book. For one thing, you couldn't bend your arms, and for another thing, it would be too hard to concentrate. I decided to bring a book on tape. Ginger offered her assistance.

"Would you like me to get this started?"

I had already set up the tape player and had it ready to go, "Yes, please. Just hit play."

Looking over the buttons on the tape player she spied the jacket of my audio book—*The Da Vinci Code*.

"I've heard that's supposed to be pretty good. It was a good idea to bring it in."

"I figured I had to do something, and I knew I would never get around to reading it. Ted told me how good it is. He enjoyed it. It's something we'll be able to talk about later. I hope it will keep my attention."

Ginger hit play and I closed my eyes. CSM churned in the background as I heard a dramatic musical overture and then... a captivating man's voice, "Random House Audio presents—*The Da Vinci Code* by Dan Brown, read for you by Colin Stinton. Louvre Museum, Paris, 10:46 P.M. Renowned curator Jaques Sauniere staggered through the vaulted archway of the museum's Grand Gallery." Colin's urgent, deep, trance-like voice was soothing, and soon became a background noise...

Teddy spun out in his socks on the linoleum floor. Beep Beep...the chase was on. He chased me from the kitchen, through the middle room, through the living room, through the dining room and back to the kitchen—a complete circle. I banged my hip on the hardwood desk in the middle room and stubbed my toe on Dolly's Barbie doll. I crashed into the old-fashioned, white porcelain sink and he put me in a half nelson. He'd rather work up a sweat chasing me than do work in the kitchen.

"Make me a banana split and I'll let you go."

"I promise. I promise."

With my fingers crossed, behind my back, I promised to make him the split. As soon as he released me, I took off for my bedroom—running up the back staircase and slamming the door. I couldn't lock it. He came thundering and stomping up the stairs. I was breathing heavily when I flung myself over the far edge of my bed and landed on the floor. He barged into my room huffing and puffing, "Fee Fi Fo Fum. I smell the blood of an Englishman. Be he alive or be he dead. I'll grind his bones to make my bread!"

I squealed in anticipation. With the quickness of a lion, he pounced on my bed and reached over the sides, digging his claws into my sides. This was the dreaded tickle torture.

"Stop it. You're hurting me."

Pinned between the wall and my bed, I had no way out. Thrashing my arms, I whacked my funny bone on the corner of the window frame. It started to tingle. He was tickling me to death. At the same time I was laughing, I was crying out for mercy.

"Stoppppppppppp!!!!!!!" I kicked the leg of my bed.

He was firm, "Not until you promise to make me a banana split."

I had to give in, "All right. All right. I promise."

Ginger squeezed her whole body in beside my bed and reached up to check the tubes. "How are you feeling?" Fortunately, I could report that I was feeling just fine. About this time, a team of doctors in their white lab coats came gliding in, clipboards in hand, looking like an episode from Doctors R Us. I could only imagine how many times Ted had lived through this scene over the past painful months. Needles and blood, needles and blood, needles and blood. It was endless. The young, female doctor with the long, brown hair and brown, suede skirt spoke up first, "You're donating for your brother, aren't you? Isn't he Ted Clark?" Nodding, it made me feel good that she remembered my brother. "He was in pretty tough shape when his wife brought him in the other day. We had some anxious moments."

"*Anxious moments*," I guess that's one way of putting it. She wasn't the only one to comment on Ted's condition the day he arrived at MGH to begin the stem cell transplant process. Several of the nurses in the Donor Center had that same "What a shame" expression. They dropped their voices a notch when they spoke about Ted lying on a hospital bed. His vital signs were abysmal. Having seen him just before this, the image was clear to me. His white skin, labored breath, fearful eyes, trembling lips, and shaking limbs were still fresh in my mind. Ted was one scared cat.

The lead doctor assured me that I would be in and out in no time. He was confident, explaining that in most cases (but Ted's was never a "most cases" scenario) donors are able to give the necessary amount of stem cells in one day. Just then, the lab technologist, Seth, came walking by. Overhearing the lead doctor, he interjected, "No, I think she's going to be in longer than one day, at least two and possibly three. We need five million."

"Oh?" the lead doctor inquired, "Why is that?"

"According to the patient's condition, and body weight, they want five million to be on the safe side."

Then, like Gandalf, Seth, the wizard of stem cells, was gone. I wanted to believe the lead doctor, but Seth had more information about

Ted's case. He was right. I was told to count on two days and be prepared for three.

"Whoaaaaa, Whoaaaaaaa!!!!!!!!" I was screaming so loud the cows in the milking parlor could hear me. Cinnamon, the mammoth four-legged female horse, was deaf to my cries. I had the reins, but no control, as we galloped down the old Dearborn Road by the farm pond. Kathy was on the saddle in back of me, and had a death grip around my waist. The faster Cinnamon galloped, the more Kathy slid. I was picturing her finally falling off—a five-foot drop, going at twenty miles per hour—onto the dirt. I was afraid she would get trampled and kicked in the head. "Whoaaaaa, Whoaaaaa!!!" My fingers were getting sore and no matter how hard I pulled on the leather strap, Cinnamon would not stop. My arms felt like they were going to rip off. Trees, decked out in their finest green leaves, flashed by me—so did my life. "Whoaaaa, Whoaaa!!!!" I was afraid I would lose my voice before I could get her to stop.

A skittish rabbit zig-zagged in front of Cinnamon and she pulled up short. Kathy hit me in the back of the head. Clunk. Cinnamon stopped galloping and dropped her massive head, flipping it from side to side. Shaking, Kathy and I climbed off her golden, red back. As I was trying to figure out what to do next, Cinnamon stepped on my foot. "Owwwwww!!!" She must have weighed a ton. I felt it all come down on my right foot. I pushed on her muscular shoulder with all the strength of a thirteen-year-old girl. It was like pushing a boulder. Where was Teddy when I needed him?

I pounded with both fists on Cinnamon's body until she lifted her hoof off my foot. I shook out the pain, vowing never to get on her again. "Kathy, we'll have to walk her back to the barn. I'm not getting back on her." Working to turn her around, I could hear clomping in the distance.

Dust was flying, as a rider and his horse grew from a blur to a shape, to a Teddy and Smokey. Teddy, the experienced rider, had mounted Smokey and led us down Dearborn Road. The black and white Smokey was much smaller than Cinnamon, and much faster. No one told us that wherever Smokey went, Cinnamon would follow. As soon as Smokey and Teddy hit the dirt road, they took off and Cinnamon did the same. Teddy fit comfortably in the saddle. Kathy and I looked like a couple of rag dolls on a coin operated hobby horse. He never looked back until he realized we were not behind him. He was a half a mile out of sight when he decided to turn around. Maybe the wind carried my voice. When Teddy got close enough, I could see this was just another playful outing for him. Invigorated from the outburst of energy, Teddy's hair was matted to his head, and his white t-shirt was plastered to his chest. His dungarees were covered in dirt. In one quick motion, he threw his leg over the side of Smokey and held onto the reins. He walked over to the three of us—a horse with no clue and two clueless riders.

"What's the problem?"

"This stupid horse took off and I couldn't get her to stop."

"Didn't you pull on the reins with both hands?"

"Duh, I pulled on the reins, but it didn't do any good."

He examined the bit, "It looks like it wasn't placed in there correctly. When you were pulling, she probably didn't feel much of anything."

"That's great to know now."

He fixed the bit, "Why don't you try again."

"I'm not getting on her again. What are you crazy? Kathy almost fell off the side of her."

"Well, Smokey's not ready to go back. He needs a good workout."

"You do what you want, but we're not getting back on her."

As we moved in the direction of the barn, I watched Teddy get back on Smokey. Jamming his left foot in the stirrup and throwing his right leg over the saddle, he plunked himself down. A black bird flying overhead dropped its green and white gooey contents on Teddy's uncapped head. Like a cracked egg, it spread down his forehead and over his ear. Teddy liked to pretend he was doing that to me with a fake egg on my head. He brushed the mess off with his bare hand and kept on going. With ease, he guided Smokey to the side of the road, across the rain-soaked gully, and up the ski hill. The ski hill was now covered in clumps of tall green grass and yellow weeds. Gone was the white snow of winter. Fearless, he let Smokey blow off some steam. Mucous sprayed from the horse's nostrils. Smokey kicked up his hind legs, and they bolted to the tree line at the top of the hill. I wished I could have done that.

I heard voices and opened my eyes. Mom was whispering with the nurse, not wanting to wake me up. She had walked around Boston and done a little shopping.

"It's all right. I'm awake."

"Would you like something to eat? I brought you a tuna fish sandwich."

I knew I needed nourishment and nibbled at the bread. Ginger came over with a carton of milk and strongly encouraged me to drink it all. When giving super cells, milk is VERY important to consume. It replaces calcium lost during the collection process.

The cold white liquid tasted good as it slid down my esophagus and coated my stomach—even though it wasn't like the farm milk. We always had plenty of milk. When Ted and I got old enough to drive, we were asked to take the car and "get some milk at the farm." We carried a three gallon tin bucket and filled it up in the milk room. There was a coffee can in the parlor for the money. It was a novelty at first but that grew old. "You go. I went the last time." "No sah. It's your turn." Eventually, I'd end up going and he'd warn me on the way out the door. "Don't spill the milk in the car." Being confined to a car with the odor of rancid, spilled milk is like walking into a closed off room where vomit hasn't been cleaned off the carpet. It just plain stinks.

Ginger was equally meticulous at the end of the day as she was at the beginning. She took away all the attached apparatus, making sure everything was done in the proper sequence. I watched as she concentrated on each step. Carefully, she pulled the needle away from my right arm. She stepped around my bed and repeated the procedure on my left.

"So how do you like this job so far?"

"It has a lot to it, but I like it. There's so much to learn."

"Well, you seem to have done a good job as far as I'm concerned. I hope this works out for you."

Leaving Ginger that afternoon, I thought about the huge responsibility she had. It wasn't a job I would like to have.

Subject: Wednesday Update
From: Muffy Faucher
Date: Wed, 24 Mar 2004

Hi family, Dave called Teddy's room at 2:15 and Jim, Mom, and Cindy were all in the room visiting. Cindy had already given her "super cells" (as she calls them) and they were waiting for an accurate counting of the cells to see if she had to come back to give more. Hopefully, she was able to give enough today. I will fill in more details as I find out. I'm actually home sick with a stomach thing. I went out to

eat at the Hanover Inn last night with an eccentric old friend. She convinced me to "try the lamb" so I did, but I wish I hadn't. That's all I saw and felt was the lamb, and it wasn't even Pamper.
(Pamper was the name of one of our childhood lambs who eventually landed on our plates.)

Dr. Small Hands called me that night and told me they needed more cells. I had not given enough. I was nauseous from the ride home. Jim, I love him dearly, is not the best driver. It's bad enough that he jams on the brakes in stop and go traffic, but he never stops talking on his cell phone. By the time he pulled around the corner by the stone wall and stopped in front of the big rock at the end of the driveway, I was ready to barf. Meekly, I opened the car door and hung my head over the tar. Nothing came up.

"Cindy, are you okay?" Jim asked.

"Yeah. Thanks, Jim. I think I'll have Debbie drive tomorrow." I was teasing him, but I was serious.

"I'm sorry. Did my driving make you sick?"

"No, sweetie. But I don't think it helped..."

I went to bed early, didn't eat a thing for supper, and got ready for day two. Between getting up at 4:30 AM on day one, not getting much sleep the previous night, lying in a Donor Center for six hours, and another fitful night, I was sick to my stomach when I woke up. I hoped taking a shower, dressing, and putting on make-up would make me feel better. (Whoever said it is better to look good than to feel good is full of shit.) I certainly couldn't roll over in bed and pull the covers over my head. The show had to go on. With water and crackers in my belly, I drove to Boston with Debbie and Mom. Debbie is a step-up from Jim, but not by much. I presented my passport to the admitting clerk.

"How are you feeling today, Mrs. Marcoux?"

"Rotten, if you really want to know." There was no "so-so" about it, I felt rotten and couldn't hide it. I am an honest person. If you don't believe me, I'll tell you. Anyone that knows me knows that I couldn't fake this. The clerk would know by looking at my face that something was wrong.

"I'll take your temperature."

"I'm fine, really, my stomach is queasy, but I know I don't have a fever." Yesterday it was the toothache, today it was the nausea. Once again, they checked me all over and determined that I was acceptable to undergo the stem cell collection.

Same as yesterday; it started with two shots of Neupogen—one 480 mg and the other 300 mg. They did STAT blood work to determine my platelet count, and hooked me up to CSM. Ginger was with me again.

"How far did you get in the book?"

"I guess about a quarter of the way through."

"Was it good?"

"I drifted some, but what I heard was good."

"Do you want me to start it for you?"

"Sure."

I watched in awe, as bright red blood traveled across my chest—one tube taking away, and one tube returning—as I listened to Colin. (The sight of something that was supposed to be on the inside, and was now on the outside of me, was puzzling.) His mesmerizing voice picked up where he had left off the day before, and again I closed my eyes.

"Just jump." I heard Teddy command, standing a few feet away.

Teetering on the hay-covered edge of the second floor of the barn, I prepared to jump off. It was a ten foot drop onto a cement floor. With my right hand, I held the thick, burly rope and kept it from swinging. With my left hand, I grabbed a hold of the noose, steadying it for my foot.

"I'm not ready yet." I let go of the rope. I chickened out.

"Bawk, bawk, buck, buck, buck, bawk..." Mimicking a chicken, Teddy climbed down the ladder to retrieve the rope. I watched him walk past the watering troughs and wade through the scattered hay. Heifers were sloppily chewing on their noon-day meal. The young female cows were tethered to the wall, covered in spider webs, facing the barn yard outside. A gentle breeze blew a black and yellow butterfly through the open window. The milk cows, standing in a line, were locked in metal yolks facing the inside of the barn. They had enough space to move their heads from side to side and up and down but not too far. I heard the flick flick of cows' tails flicking away black flies. Munching on hay, one of the cows raised his head as Teddy walked by. He rubbed the white splotch on the bridge of the protruding nose, and black, marble-like cow's eyes followed him to the rope. I inhaled the sweet smell of hay, mingled with cow manure. Mom, a farmer's daughter, taught me to love that smell. Teddy grabbed the rope, hanging from the center, supporting beam in the middle of the barn, and yelled from down below, "Catch this."

The trick was to stand close enough to catch the rope, but not close enough to fall off the edge. Sometimes it took two or three times before I could catch it, because it may be just out-of-reach or fly too far over my head. Sometimes it would bonk me on the head on the way back down. It always made me a little nervous. Teddy pulled back on the rope and gave it a heave. The rope curled and sailed through the air like the cows' swishing tails. Its heavy knot, part way up, followed the noose at the end. I reached out and grabbed it.

"Good. Now wait until I get back up there."

I held the knot in the rope and tried to push the knot in my stomach down. I really wanted to jump. Teddy came around in back of me, and held me by my t-shirt.

"I won't let you fall. You can do this."

He steadied me while I struggled to get my foot in the noose. It's a bit like taking off on one ski in shallow water. The timing has to be just right. Balancing on the supporting foot and pushing down on the other would propel me forward. Once I got my foot in the noose, I knew it was best to jump immediately. That way, I could make sure I was clear away from the edge and wouldn't accidentally hit the wooden support beam. It was also like diving far enough out from the high diving board so you wouldn't hit the lower one. Taking a deep breath, I grabbed the rope as hard as I could and jumped.

Air rushed by me and my left foot snuggled into the noose. My toes pinched me as I straightened out my knee. I hugged the rope and let it swing me in mid-air. The downward force made my stomach sink; and being afflicted with motion sickness, it made me feel queasy. I swirled through the crack in the huge, open barn doors. I twirled with the rope. I was dangling from the rafters! In seconds, I was back at the edge of the second floor.

Ginger, diligently charting, was on the other side of the room when my upset stomach sent off a final warning signal. It had been warning me all morning—gurgling and flipping its contents. The little amount that I had in it, was about to come flying out. I yelled to her, "Ginger." She looked up from my medical chart, saw my cheeks bulging, and ran for a basin. She stuck it under my chin in time to catch the gross gastric juices and chunks of undigested crackers. When she cleaned my lips with a warm wash cloth she asked, "What did you eat last night?"

"Not much. I felt too lousy too eat. And...I got car sick on the way home."

"We'll get you some Compazine for your ride tonight and we'll need to increase your calcium intake. We'll double up on that tomorrow. Sorry about that. Is there anything I can get for you now?"

"No. I feel much better all ready."

She readjusted the pillow under my elbow and fluffed the pillows under my neck.

"I guess I'll have to keep a closer eye on you."

At the end of the day, as Ginger pulled the needle out of my right arm, Mom and Debbie walked to the foot of my bed. They had returned from a long day of walking.

"Hey, Cindy," Debbie asked, "How are you?"

She glanced over the tubing and contraptions, and flinched at the sight of my arm. Debbie's ability to take everything in stride was being tested. In a pinch, I could always count on Debbie to remain cool, calm, and collected. Yet, this ordeal was even taking the quickness out of Debbie's usual fast pace. She asked with apprehension, "Did you want to see Ted when you're all done here?"

"No. I think I'll pass. I don't think I can take the elevator today. You and Mom can go up and visit him now and give him my love."

As she and Mom left the room, Debbie wasn't smiling, "I hope you feel better. We'll be back soon to get you."

That night, in the quiet of my den, I wrote the following email:

Subject: One More to Go
Hi all,

Well, two days down and one to go. Dr. Small Hands just called and politely requested my presence back at the donor center tomorrow. I guess they just didn't get enough of those super cells yet! (At this point they had collected 3.4 million CD 34 stem cells.) They did start giving Ted the cells that were collected yesterday. I spoke with him around 5:00 P.M. and he sounded good. He was disappointed that he couldn't get on the bike because his platelet count was too low. He didn't get quite as good a night sleep because he kept having to get up to use the bathroom and he was having some nausea this morning. That makes two of us. Nothing like getting some drugs to calm that down...right, Ted!!! (The Compazine worked well for me.)

I know you have been having a chuckle at my expense because when Ted is converted to my blood he will have trouble with the following: using a remote control, having anyone touch his ears, developing migraines, etc., etc. But, have you thought about the good things...like...he will be one hell of a dancer!! Tomorrow's schedule – Jim is bringing me in and Brenda is bringing me home.
Love to all,
The Donor

Muffy wrote back to me:

Hi Donor, I'm proud of you, Cindy. I know it hasn't been easy. Love, Muf

TGIF was in the air, Friday March 26th—day three. Black Hawk was in charge of me today. (She did have kind of a military presence.) She had watched me come and go on the two previous days, and I knew she had followed me every cell of the way. Ginger had the day off, and I missed seeing her. Black Hawk pulled up a chair, sat by my bed, and took the time to chat. It felt like old home week.

"You back again?' she joked, "This is a first. We never see anyone more than two days in a row."

"Yeah. I had so much fun the last two days I had to come back for some more."

"You going to finish that book?"

"I don't know, we'll see."

"How's that stomach today?"

"Much better. Much, much better!"

She looked over my left arm without gasping, gently turning it from side to side. The huge, purple and blue bruise, in the middle of my arm, was becoming quite noticeable. The interim tech didn't do such a good job the day before.

"Does it hurt?"

"No. It just looks bad."

She made sure there were no lumps or swelling, "We'll put the returning needle—the smaller one—in this side, and try to stay away from yesterday's hole."

"That's a wonderful idea."

In the same manner as Ginger, after Black Hawk got me set up, propped up, and CSM was running, she started my tape. "Sophie

Neveu, despite working in law enforcement, had never found herself at gunpoint until tonight…"

In the sterile, hospital room enshrined in white—white sheets, white walls, white gloves, and white skin—the conversation Ted and I have again and again begins.

"Hi, Ted, how are you feelin'?"

"Not too bad."

"Would you like me to rub your feet?' I took my cue from Becky.

"Sure." The answer was always, "Yes."

He shifted under the sheets lifting his butt; the flabby, limp skin fell over a bony form that once was a robust asset. Surely, it was bedsore-bound. He grabbed the bed rails to hoist himself up and made his feet accessible. I scooped under the mattress and pulled the blankets away, uncovering both colorless feet. (The hair on his toes had already fallen out.) They were puffy and swollen and looked like they hurt but he didn't complain.

In the top drawer of his bedside table, I found the pink bottle of baby lotion, and squeezed a big glob into my hands. The smell made me think of changing my baby's diapers. I made sure I had plenty to work with. First I'd do the left and then I'd do the right. I started in the bottom, right corner of his arch and pressed my thumbs up along the curve of his foot. Reaching the plateau, where the foot spreads out, I used both hands to massage and caress. I thumbed my way back down, pushing in along the arch until I reached his heel. By then, I needed more cream to cover his heel—dry from lack of use, dry from lying in pressurized air, and dry from being treated with chemicals.

I could sense his body relaxing. He rested the back of his head on his pillow, and closed his eyes.

"Sorry I'm not such good company." I could barely hear Ted's words.

"It's okay to go to sleep." I whispered back to him from the foot of his bed.

Listening to my tape with my eyes wide open, I saw Seth enter the Donor Center. He made me smile. He came by to check how things were going, and I had a chance to ask him some questions.

"How many more cells do you need?"

"The miracle number for today is one point six million."

"What if I don't get to one point six million?"

"Well, we already have a good supply. We'll be able to use what we have. It's just that in Ted's case, they want to be sure to have an extra good amount."

"Would they let me come back tomorrow?"

"No way." He shook his head side to side. "Your platelet count is getting too low. There is no way they would let you come in again that soon."

At the end of day three, I felt euphoric. It was probably due to the relief that my part was over. Jimmy and Brenda met me in the Donor Center and we devoured some free pizza. I even felt well enough to travel the fourteen floors in the elevator, holding my stomach on each stop.

Ted was smiling when we trooped in, "Hey, CC. Thanks for your super cells."

"You're very welcome. After all the grief you've given me, you're a lucky guy."

"I know."

We made a quick visit. It was getting near rush hour and we wanted to beat the traffic. I looked at him closely before saying my last good-bye. My voice started to quake, "I love you, man. Hang in there, and let my super cells get to work." He put up both thumbs, "I will."

It was Jimmy's turn to email the family.

Subject: Ted 3/26/04
From: Jim Clark
Hi All:
My turn to communicate:

Well it is now official. Ted is a he/she. He now has the XX chromosome makeup and not the XY anymore. Cindy has transformed the big guy. Ted is B+ and not B-, but who cares as long as he doesn't wear high heels and lipstick.

Cindy was in rare form today acting her normal giddy self, laughing about nothing in particular. She was giggling so hard I thought she would wet the bed, and she would blame it on me for making her laugh, and then I would have to clean it up. I mean, what is so funny about me slipping on the ice when I was getting gas on Wednesday? She didn't even see me slip. All I did was tell her about it. But now she remembers that I had snow all over my jacket when I got in the car. That was all it took. Jog her memory, and its off to the giggle races!

Today was a very good day. Cindy had her last apheresis for Ted. The goal today was to collect 1.6 million CD 34 stem cells. For the 3 days they wanted to collect 5 million stem cells. We will know tonight how much she gave officially. Cindy was feeling much better today. My driving today did not make her sick. We left at 5:30 and got home at 5:00 pm Brenda was also in today.

Ted looks great and was not nauseous when I was there. He wanted to get on his bike, but couldn't until his platelets get over 20 (17 now). Ted is scheduled to get the remaining stem cells at 6:00 pm tonight.

Jim

I was snoozing on my living room couch, about ready to fall asleep, when the phone rang.

"Hello, this is Dr. Miles."

"Hi."

"I wanted to let you know we collected over five million stem cells."

Gulping down tears I managed to say, "Thank you so much."

Day is Done

    Boris, our fifteen-pound Maine Coon cat, climbed on my back. He started kneading me in the neck like I was a ball of dough. He always goes for the jugular. I've tried to train him to get the kink out of my left shoulder blade, but he's not very trainable. Repeatedly, in a circular motion, his paws dug into my skin. Occasionally, I felt a sharp toenail. I pushed him away with one hand, and placed my other hand on my neck as protection. He wouldn't leave me alone. Lightly, he placed one paw on my bare shoulder. I opened my eyes and his green and black eyes were staring at me. Like a child that appears at your bedside and breathes warm air on your face, he is irresistible. As I scratched under his chin he tilted his head back and started grooving, purring for more. I massaged the crevice between his right ear and the top of his head.

    Boris's markings are that of a ferocious cat. The tuft of fur under his neck is black, white, and gray, and forms the shape of a royal mane. Two thick black lines start at the corners of his eyes and dip down into his velvety fur. Other black streaks line his forehead. His ears are pointed, and he pulls them back when he is ready to pounce. White, spindly whiskers tickle my nose and distinguish him as master of his domain. We let him walk all over us. When he squints, he looks like a lion—king of the forest. As he prowls across my bed and leaps into the window, I decide it is time to get up. It is 6:00 AM on Memorial Day, May 29, 2006.

    I told Mom I would meet her at the Kensington cemetery to watch the parade. It was scheduled to start at 8:00 AM, and I wanted to ride my bike. I showered and dressed in my black biking pants and white, short sleeve shirt. Across the front of my cotton shirt is the American flag and U.S.A. in bold letters—I am proud to be an American. Only restless, gray squirrels are awake, scampering across the yard, as I lower the American flag to half mast and survey the front lawn. It is lusciously deep green. Pink and purple azaleas are fading in the garden to my left, while white and rose-colored rhododendrons in the garden to my right are bursting in bloom. Pots of yellow and red gerbera daisies flank each side of our red granite step. I see buds on our miniature weigela bushes. Recently planted white alyssum, yellow marigolds, and blue ageratum are meticulously placed in the front yard garden, between two brick paths. One path leads to the picket fence, the other to the driveway. Across the road are remnants of a stone wall and huge maple trees. Branches arch over the road. Beyond the brick path, beyond the road, and beyond the hill, I know the stand-alone tree is waiting for the sun to appear. I am blessed.

Weathermen predicted showers and it looks like it might rain as I lace up my sneakers. Boris rubs his head against my leg and whines and sniffs at my feet. No, Boris, you can't come with me. I grab the navy blue gortex jacket I bought recently to take to Iceland, and carry it to the shed to get my bike. It is a bit chilly—around fifty-five degrees. Despite the threat of raindrops, I wheel my bike across the lawn and into the driveway. There are no signs of cars as I zip up my jacket and secure my feet in the pedals. Rain or shine, I need to ride my bike.

At a leisurely pace I ride down Sanborn Road and across the railroad tracks. I turn right on Route 108 and downshift as I pedal up the steep hill toward Carmen's Diner. At the top of the hill I turn left onto Stumpfield Road—the road to the farm. I stop at my cousin Hal's to see if he is going to the parade, but he is not at home. I continue toward the farm. Riding alongside the electric fence, I look across the field. In the distance are bales of hay wrapped in white, plastic, shrink wrap and the blood-sucker infested pond. An abandoned tractor and discarded farm equipment show signs of wear and tear. I think of Teddy, out there mowing the fields on number eight hundred and twenty-six.

Subject: Ted update
Date: Sat, 3 Apr 2004

Hi everyone, Ron & I went to see Ted today. He was receiving more platelets. His count was 10. The good news is that his wbc was up to .3 (300). This is a good indication that Lucinda's super cells may be starting to work. His spleen has enlarged again but no fever this morning. He was a little nauseated but Ativan helped him eat some of his noon meal. He is bald now but still handsome. His major complaint was fatigue. He is not sleeping too well as he has to get up to urinate. This is because he has had to take a diuretic to get rid of some fluid in the lungs. His oxygen saturation was 100% when we were there. His hematocrit was 22. Pat & Lucinda were supposed to visit this afternoon. He let me give him a foot rub & he tolerated my request for him to listen to a relaxation tape of cows in an Alpine meadow. He is a good patient. Love to all, Becky

The hind ends of black and white cows were visible through the path between two large, cow barns. I rode past the red, milking barn with the open doors, past Dearborn Road, and up the steady incline. Glancing to my left, at the top of the hill, I thought about moonlit nights we used to go sledding on hard-packed snow. The view of a grass-covered meadow, sloping downhill, and ending with a row of trees is memorable. And, to think that my cousin Hal's daughter will be building a home there soon, how fortunate. I hunched over my handlebars and enjoyed the rush of not using any brakes. I didn't even wear a helmet. Near the end of Stumpfield Road I took another left onto Trundle Bed Road, and then another, bringing me to the center of Kensington.

I thought I had the time wrong. There wasn't a soul in sight. I passed the white Kensington Grange No. 173 P and the rust-colored, brick Kensington Social Library. The doors to the fire station were open, but I didn't see anyone there. I continued beside the Kensington Elementary School; and then something hit me. It came from behind the clouds. Like listening to the Star Spangled Banner at the start of Mandy's basketball games, I knew I was going to cry. Why was that?

This place was filled with peace—no traffic, no congestion, and no bombs—we are at war in Iraq. I can't say exactly what triggered the swell of emotion. But, an invisible, internal symphony reached a crescendo inside me that was impossible to ignore. Perhaps it was the beauty of an unencumbered morning; perhaps it was the memories ever-present on my mind, perhaps the acknowledgement of feeling blessed, and the sadness for those who are not. Perhaps, it was a little of pre-menopausal symptoms. Whatever the cause, spontaneously, I began to cry. Tears, marching to their own beat, paraded down my cheeks. I passed a small gathering, milling around the Kensington Town Hall and I wondered if they saw me crying, but, I didn't care if they did. My nose was beginning to fill up and I didn't have any tissues—*not even a pocket handkerchief.* I rode around the back of the white, Protestant, Congregational church with black shutters. Numerous cousins, mothers, aunts, and uncles had been married here. The sign on the side of the building by the white rhododendron bush was labeled in black letters, "First Congregational Church, United Church of Christ, Established 1737." It had a traditional, pointed steeple.

I got off my bike and leaned it against the wooden frame outlining the edge of the church flower bed. My Aunt Dolly helped plant that garden. Through tear-soaked eyes, I focused on the plants. A variegated hosta was closest to me, shading the spread of violets. White, tear-shaped droplets from Solomon's seal draped over flowering perennials gone by. Scattered throughout were bleeding hearts. Aunt Dolly wanted a garden that was low maintenance. Each window box was filled with pink geraniums and one small American flag. This is a Protestant church. Nothing too showy for us. I put my hands on my hips, and my shoulders shook, as tears came gushing out.

Subject: Ted
Date: Sat. 17 Apr 2004

Hi, Sorry this is late. I spoke to Ted Friday about 4:30 pm. He was just finishing his bike ride with physical therapist. He went on about 35 min. He felt pretty good. He is hacking up a lot, probably the result of pneumonia. His wbc went down a little, his hct was about the same and his platelets went up to 44. Not sure when he will come home. Maybe Monday. Nobody was in to see him Friday. Jim

Wiping my nose with the side of my finger, I got back on my bike. Cars were starting to pull into the parking lot across from the church. A mother was holding her child's hand as they walked across the street. A car here and a car there pulled off the side of the road. I peddled back toward the fire station and the cemetery, passing the Union Meeting House/Universalist Church 1865. It was about two hundred yards from the Congregational Church.

The black, wrought iron fence surrounding the cemetery reminded me of Savannah—only this one didn't have a bird girl. Sharp points topped the sturdy metal and prohibited anyone from attempting to jump over. As I approached the gate, swung open for the morning, I caught a glimpse of a steel gray marker. Still riding my bike, one word caught my attention—DIED—large letters etched in stone. My tears runneth over. Firemen were manning the station, drinking coffee and eating doughnuts. Again I wondered, did they see me crying? I turned into the cemetery, steering my front wheel along the rut in the dirt path. With reverence, I pondered the names on the gravestones.

There were old New England first names like Mary, Eunice, Benjamin, and Wilbur. Last names were familiar too, like Palmer, Brewster, Prescott, and Moulton. How many times had Mom spoken about Moulton's Ridge? To me, it was a place, not a person. Seeing the name in writing, I made the connection. Town founders were buried everywhere. How long had it been since I was in this cemetery? I could not remember. I could not remember where my grandmother and grandfather Bodwell were buried, and I looked for their names. Along the way, I paused and read, Herbert M Jordan, PFC US Marine Corps, World War II, Jan 10, 1925 – Mar 30, 2002. I was here, on this day, to pay respect to these fallen heroes.

I continued to the back of the cemetery and leaned my bike against the brown, wooden, trash bin, labeled "trash," in white letters. It should be safe here under the trees. Alone in the cemetery, I walked between and over the mounds of grass, looking for Harold Bodwell. I saw Abbie F. wife of John Gill, 1840 – 1906, and Charles Titcomb died May 4, 1873, and John Blake and his wife Mary Philbrick. There was a Rebecca, and a Martha, and a Dorothy. A tall, spiked monument, like the Washington Memorial, was dedicated to Mr. Dearborn. I thought about the name—dear...born...--and wondered how he had made his fortune. There were two granite steps embedded in the ground leading the way to the base. I walked up the steps and stood on the grass platform, and peered at the letters: George E. Dearborn, Born in Kensington, NH April 16, 1825, Died in Philadelphia, PA May 7, 1897, At Rest. I added...Amen. How many times had I heard Mom refer to the "old Dearborn Road?" He must have been quite a guy.

Casting light over the rows of granite tomb stones, the sun began to illuminate the day. The chill of daybreak was giving way to a midmorning glow. I felt myself getting warmer. I removed my jacket and tied it around my waist. My eyes followed the contours of the markers—Lucy Warren was engraved in a white, stone heart low to the ground; Palmer was inscribed above the intricate details of an unrolled piece of parchment paper; and Jordan was in a simple, dark-gray square. As with death, these tokens came in all shapes and forms. Conscientious mourners were silently filing in, as I continued on my search. A small crowd was beginning to gather along the roadside near the fire station. I heard my name called from a distance, "Cindy." I looked toward the fence and saw Becky waving. She had on a navy blue, short-sleeved shirt with the American flag on the front.

Subject: Hi Jim
Date: Fri, 23 Apr 2004
From: Ted

Hi James
Had a nice visit from Hal, Elaine, and Melissa for a couple hours last night before they went out for supper. Hal was telling me how much Jordan enjoys the farm. Still not sure I will be able to go home. I have a mild rash, which is probably host verses graft and can't figure out what is causing a cough. I still have some fine-tuning to do yet. I'm getting the Neupogen shot which should be helping with the white cells. A good thing is I haven't had any blood transfusion in over a week.   Ted

I forgot about looking for Grandpa Bodwell's gravestone and walked back to the road. Small clusters of locals, shaking hands and hugging one another, were lining up for the parade.

"Hi, Becky. I see you're wearing an American flag, too. Good choice. Where's Mom?"

"She should be right along. She's just down the road somewhere."

"I see you have the boys."

Jason, the dark-haired, five-year-old, was holding an American flag and lightly touching Becky's thigh. Derek, the reddish/blond-haired, three-year-old, was dragging his.

"Derek, hold your flag up. You mustn't let it touch the ground," Becky said.

He looked at Becky with questioning eyes, but did as he was told.

Mom, with a bounce in her step, greeted her first and third generation off-spring—Becky and her boys. Comfortable with her age, wearing cotton top and khaki shorts, she looked marvelous. This was her stomping grounds. She was born and raised in Kensington. Mom, and the other elementary school children, made Memorial Day wreaths. Each year they gathered enough evergreen vines to wrap into a circle. The simple wreath, without any bow, was placed over their arm. Each of them carried a miniature American flag as they paraded into the cemetery. They knew to place them on a Veteran's marker.

"Great color, Mom!" Becky complimented the tangerine, short-sleeved, collared shirt. Becky's always giving her a hard time about what color she wears.

Mom puffed out her chest and arched her back proudly, "You think so?"

"Oh, yeah. That's a great color for you."

Smiling, Mom looked down at her great-grandchildren, "Would you like to see where your great, great grandfather is buried?"

The boys took off giggling and laughing, and we caught up with them in one of the rows near Charles Titcomb Died May 4, 1873.

Derek stopped on one of the mounds. With pure, unadulterated innocence he looked up at me and asked, "Why don't they unbury them?"

I let that question go unanswered. He got distracted before he thought to ask it again.

Subject: Ted update
Date: Mon, 3 May 2004

Hi Everyone, I just spoke with Ted at home!!!!! He is very glad to be out of the hospital. I asked him to email a list of foods he is allowed to have and other precautions so when we visit we will be following protocol. Counts are still low and lung complications have not resolved. He will need to go back to the clinic at MGH on Thurs. Jim plans to take him. Brenda picked him up at the hosp. She plans to go to Maine on Wed. & help Corey pack & come home for the summer. Things are looking up but please keep prayers & positive vibes headed in his direction.
Becky

Mom kept walking in the direction of the tree line, in the very back of the cemetery. I kept glancing toward the trash receptacle to make sure my bike was still there. Why didn't I remember where my grandparents' gravestone was? I was thirteen, a very unlucky number, when Grandpa Bodwell died, and I was thirty-three when Grammy died. I was old enough to remember, but for some reason I didn't. I attended both their funerals and stood in the cemetery among family and friends. I should have known where they rested in peace. My ignorance continued to bother me as I listened to Mom explain where other family members were buried, like Uncle Clark. I was at his funeral too.

"Derek, don't step there."

Mom, Becky, and I all reached to tug him away from Abraham—written on a shiny, dark blue, flat surface. It was deeply entrenched in the ground and spikes of grass surrounded it on all sides—it was hardly noticeable. Derek walked around it and ran off to catch up with Jason. Jason was pointing out the special markers that denote a fireman. His dad's a fireman.

"Mom," I asked, "Do you know how Mr. Dearborn made his money?" I pointed to the Washington Memorial.

"No. I'm not really sure. You'll have to ask Aunt Dolly."

Mom continued to guide us toward the last row of gravestones. I would not have guessed it was so far back. John Blake and his wife Mary Philbrick were in the front couple of rows. Did it make a difference? Up one knoll and down, and past a few more stones and we were getting close. Even without my glasses, I could make out the bold letters: BODWELL.

Subject: Ted
From: Jim Clark
Date: Thu, 6 May 2006

Ted and I had a long day. I picked Ted up at 8:30 am. We got into Mass General about 10:15. I dropped him off and went to Lexington to see customers so I got a lot of work done. We left Boston at 5:00 and got to Ted's house after 7:00. Ted has some good signs as follows:

WBC up to 6.4 (normal)
HCT 25? Up a little
Platelets 29 (low) but improved from 20 Monday. He had no platelet infusion Monday so this means his bone marrow is manufacturing them. Doctor says Ted spleen is smaller than 2 weeks ago and even since Friday.

Should note that Ted's counts will still fluctuate. He was told not to take Neupogen shots for now, but likely that WBC will drop again. He did have a blood infusion today which is what took much of the time. His potassium level is high. His sodium and magnesium is low. This has to do with his meds. He is a little shaky. He is drinking a lot as he should but water may be flushing some of sodium out. Maybe some Gatorade and Propel will help. Ted says he will eat some potato chips. I only provided this info cause I was present and I know Ted probably doesn't want this all the time. Looks like the days he will go in are Mondays and Thursdays at 10:30.

*Monday 5/10 Brenda will transport him in
Thursday 5/13 Not determined, but I can do it*

*Mom will make a schedule.
Jim*

    The rectangular, dark gray granite was firmly set in the ground, variegated hostas on each side. Aunt Dolly, who again did the planting, likes her hosta. Decorating the front was a flower box filled with pink geraniums and dainty white trailing annuals. And, she likes her pink geranium. It was a modest, yet substantial stone, weighing close to a ton. It was approximately three feet wide and four feet high. I had to walk around the back and under draping tree limbs to read the inscription: Harold W Bodwell 1905 – 1969, his wife Dorothy C Turner 1906 – 1989. Grandpa Bodwell was the one who started the farm. How many stories has Mom told me about her days on the farm? "Why…I used to spray my school books with perfume so my classmates wouldn't know I'd been milking the cows before school." Grandpa's son was named Harold W. Bodwell, Junior, and he worked on the farm. "Junior" had to leave the farm when he served in World War II—when he returned he wasn't called "Junior" any more.

    "You know," my Mom pointed out, "Uncle Harry was stationed in Bora Bora during the war." And, Hal, Harold W. Bodwell, III, continues to manage the farm. "Hal came back from New York to help Uncle Harry with the farm." Unimpressed, Jason took a five-year-old's look at the marker and scurried into the woods. Derek was right behind him. I slapped a mosquito and wondered if the boys were sprayed with repellent.

    Becky trampled into the woods after them, "Come on, Jason. Come on, Derek. Come out of the woods. Let's see if the parade is getting started." She got Jason by his hand and escorted him out.

Turning away from the stone, Mom and I started over the mounds. The sun was warming the grounds and it was starting to get hot. Perhaps it wasn't going to rain after all. I saw Aunt Dolly. Her distinguished, straight, dark gray hair was cut short. She was dressed in casual walking pants and a blue cotton top. Nothing too flashy for her. Aunt Dolly's hunched over gait is similar to Mom's. People of Exeter get them confused. I recognize her immediately. As sure as there are remains buried beneath me, there is Yankee in her bones.

"Hi, Aunt Dolly." I asked, "Do you know how Mr. Dearborn made his money?"

I listened to a brief history about where the house was, who lived there, how the house burned, and then Aunt Dolly turned to me and confessed, "I really don't know how he made his money."

Unsuccessful with that, I decided to ask her about Iceland. I was traveling to Iceland the coming weekend to meet up with Pat on his return from a business trip in Norway. Mom kept telling me to ask Aunt Dolly about it because her husband, Buzz, was stationed there during the war.

"What should I know about Iceland? I've been having troubling trying to establish distances between the main sight-seeing features."

Honestly, she answered, "You should ask Buzz about that, he'd be able to give you the best information."

I took her at her word, "Thanks, Aunt Dolly. I will."

She left it at, "Buzz is having coffee in the fire station."

Subject: Ted update
Date: Mon, 17 May 2004

Sorry to report that Ted is back at MGH. He had a regular MD appt. today & they decided to admit him. As you all know he has not been feeling too well & needs medical evaluation. He has been running fevers again & probably needs hydration along with blood tests. Hopefully, it will be a short stay. We will post the room & telephone number as soon as we know. He will be back on the same floor.
Becky

I looked both ways, even though there was little chance of any cars coming, and walked across the street. Becky, the boys, and Mom found other interests. With a cup of coffee in one hand and a plain, old-fashioned doughnut in the other, Buzz was guarding the refreshment table. He was wearing fireman's attire: a gray shirt with Kensington Fire Department and navy blue pants. He was firmly planted on stable ground. Like Ted, Buzz is not known to be a talker, unless he has something to say. He does not use words when they are unsolicited; he uses them when they are needed. Buzz did a nice job refinishing an old chair of mine. That's what he likes to do. I never had more than a couple sentence conversation with him. Mom took care of the exchanges. Now, I had something specific to ask him.

"Hi, Buzz. I heard you were stationed in Iceland, and you and Aunt Dolly visited there recently. I'm leaving this Friday and wanted to pick your brains. Do you think the Blue Lagoon is worth it?"

Buzz smiled and licked his lips, "Oh sure. When they built the power plant all this water collected in a big pool. These people started swimming in it and discovered that it cleared up their skin problems. After that it became a real attraction. It has this volcanic mud around the edges and that's kind of cool." He looked across the street and laughed, refreshing his memory, "Dolly swam in it."

"We're staying at the Hotel Loftleider. They told me we could walk to town from there but I can't seem to visualize what that would look like because of the odd terrain there."

"You can walk it." He paused and took a bite of his doughnut, trying to recreate a picture for me, "Up the hill from that hotel is a beautiful view…that's a good place to be. We went on one of the tours that took us around to see the hot springs and the waterfall." Other informed travelers may have said, "You'll have to do that, or don't miss such and such," but Buzz just recited what he had seen and done. I liked his style.

"Did you go on the Golden Circle Tour? I've heard that is the main one."

Buzz nodded and took another swig of his coffee. "When we flew in at night the lights were incredible. Not like when I was there during the war. There was only one street when I was there." He shook his head and drifted.

Glancing down the street, I heard the Exeter High School Band. Nudging my way out from under the roof, I smiled while Buzz continued to talk. "There's plenty to see there." I wanted to be on the other side of the street before the front of the parade got to the fire station, and I had to cut him off. "Thanks, Buzz. I feel better about what to expect. Thanks again, I have to go…" Crossing the street, I glanced back over my shoulder; I saw Buzz smiling to himself—he was still in Iceland.

Subject: Ted
Date: Wed., 26 May 2004

Ted did not go home today—I guess that the Drs. wanted to be sure the oral meds. he will be taking at home will work o.k. as they are replacing the IV ones he has been having. Of course he was disappointed but has been told he can go at 10:00 tomorrow, Brenda will get him. On Friday Dave plans to take him in for his appt. at the clinic at M.G.H. Let us hope that nothing prevents him from getting home tomorrow and that all goes well from now on. Such a long struggle, so much courage to hang in!! What a guy!! We all do love him so!!! Love, Mom

I saw the back of Hal's white, preppy-like, collared shirt (he does clean up well), and crept up on him. He was chatting with Becky, leaning against the black Savannah fence. I poked him in the side, forcing him to spin around.

"Hey!" I tried to look annoyed, "I have a bone to pick with you."

"What?" He looked as innocent as Derek dragging his American flag.

"What's this I hear about Sarah?"

A "proud as a newly informed father that he is going to be a grandfather" smile spread across his face, "Sarah's pregnant." He consented to give his daughter's hand in marriage with the promise of grandchildren. At her wedding, they danced to "She thinks my tractor's sexy." And, Sarah's grandfather made the toast, saying, "As the Bible says, go forth and multiply." Children were definitely in her future.

"I know… and I have to hear it from my mom, not from the horse's mouth. I would have expected a call from you. What's the deal?"

He tried to justify the oversight, "Well, we weren't even sure when we were supposed to tell people. She had some trouble at first." He grew a tad serious.

"I know. I heard about that, too. I'll let you off the hook this time."

The parade marshals, holding the long, rectangular banner, were almost parallel to us. The rat-tat-tats of drum sticks were clearly heard. We turned our attention to the marchers. Hal took out his camera and got ready to take a picture of his dad—Harold Bodwell, Junior—still able to fit in his WWII uniform. He was approaching eighty years old. Walking slowly with his comrades to the other side of him, Uncle Harry looked our way. He smiled, and then, like the number of years behind him, it vanished. The smile was to recognize the people he knew, its fading was to recognize those that were not with us. Long hours under the heat of the sun, driving tractors and bailing hay, aged and wrinkled his face. He did not smile again, as the parade continued on... and Hal snapped a picture.

From: Patrick Marcoux
To: Ted & Brenda
Sent: Monday, May 31, 2004
Subject: Pictures

Lucy is cruising

Attached to the email were pictures of me—my first attempt at roller skating with my new blue sparkly sketchers. (I picked them up for $20.00—they were hard to resist.) I was wearing knee pads, elbow pads, protective gloves and a helmet, looking as shaky and nervous as my four-year-old granddaughter with her first pair of roller blades. Pat captured me swerving my way down the slope in front of our house—it was big and it went downhill—but it wasn't a big downhill. I know Ted chuckled when he saw the pictures.

Subject: Re: pictures
From: Ted Clark
Date: Tue, 1 June 2004

Nice pictures, I didn't know that Lucy was a hockey blade cruiser. She looks like she needs a team to play on. I'd like to see her make it down the farm hill. Ted

The marshals turned the corner and made their way into the cemetery, the politicians in a polished black car, the jump ropers and the wee band of baseball players trailing after them. Six-year-olds, in their clean, navy blue shirts with white team lettering, made me think of Teddy and Skippy. Kingston's Babe Ruther's used to march in our Memorial Day parade. (The picture of Teddy and Skippy in their little league uniforms—Ted leaning on his baseball bat, came to mind.) I watched as one brown-haired boy joked around and jabbed a blond-haired boy in the ribs—laughing at something in their sight.

A red Kensington fire truck eased by the gathering and a young, curly, blond-haired girl sat proudly in the front seat. Her face just barely appeared in the window. She waved to onlookers, as her dad held one hand on the steering wheel and rested his elbow on the window frame. The Exeter High School marching band, made its way down the street. Dressed in blue and white uniforms, these teenagers filled in the gaps. The Kensington parade was supposed to start at 8:00 AM because the sought-after band was due in other parades. Long blond strands hung from under the hat of one of the trumpeters, and a black ponytail accompanied a flute player—they followed their leader and entered the hallowed grounds.

The Big Day—as Mom would put it—was June 19, 2004. It was the Bodwell family reunion and this year, it was held at "cousin Hal's," just up from the farm. Over one hundred relatives from as close as Kensington to as far as California were gathered to renew family ties. Standing on Hal's front lawn, with notes in hand, Aunt Dolly made an announcement:

"Once again we reunite in celebration of our proud heritage of family. The wonderful booklet Peggy Jo Adams put together for our 2002 reunion in Vermont gave us a glimpse into the lives of our more ancient ancestors. Many of us have copies of Uncle Joe's "Gramps" memoir, written at the request of his children, which of course included many stories of the whole family of Willard and Carrie Gage Bodwell. This memoir is a treasure as it gives my generation of cousins a brief look into the lives of our parents. It is a good thing to think back to a time gone by and have this insight and understanding of events that have indeed shaped our lives and brought us to gather here today."

And with that, the younger generation came forward to act out their parts in the Bodwell family skit. Jordan was Joseph, Tyler was Ralphie, and Jillian was Ruthie. They reenacted a summer night about the Bodwell's arrival in Kensington. The history started with Willard Bodwell and Carrie Cage who married in Methuen, MA in August of 1882. How Mom and Aunt Dolly got these kids, in 2004, to act in a family play was beyond me. I laughed as Jordan climbed on the antique tractor with Hal and…Ted entered the scene.

The walking dead man, step by step, made his way across the driveway and began to mingle with the crowd. Those that had only heard, but had not seen, must have been shocked. Whispered words passed from ear to ear after he passed by. I was concerned if he had eaten, "Ted, can I get you a hamburger?" He answered politely, "Sure." He was withered, weak, and pale, wearing his familiar baseball hat as he stopped to chat with Skippy and Hal. I went to the grill to fix him a hamburger and returned to catch the three of them in days gone by, "Remember when we…" Skippy could always get Teddy to laugh.

As hard as it must have been, Ted made the effort to get there—it was his last day on the farm.

A transparent veil of silence spread over the solemn crowd—the master of ceremonies announced that a poem would be read by one of the younger generation. A poised eleven-year-old stood in front of the crowd, and held a microphone to his mouth.

He eloquently recited:

In Flanders Fields
John Mc Crae (1872 – 1918)

In Flanders Fields the poppies blow
Between the crosses, row on row
That mark our place; and in the sky
The larks, still bravely singing, fly
Scarce heard amid the guns below.

We are the dead. Short days ago
We lived, felt dawn, saw sunset glow,
Loved and were loved, and now we lie
In Flanders fields.

Take up our quarrel with the foe:
To you from failing hands we throw
The torch: be yours to hold it high.
If ye break faith with us who die
We shall not sleep, though poppies grow
In Flanders fields.

What this meager group of marchers and spectators lacked in numbers they made up for in character—it carried the day. They were respectful, purposeful community members, commemorating the dead. Little ones were hushed as parents stood at attention. I clasped my hands in front of me and Dad lowered his head as the master of ceremonies continued.

"We are gathered here to pay our respects to the many heroes who have led our nation and committed their lives to making our country a better place to live."

From the gate swung open, down the dirt path, across the mounds of grass, and under the spreading oak tree, people stopped what they were doing. Wherever they were in the cemetery they stood still. A tall, composed young woman with short blond hair and blue eyes smiled as she united with a familiar friend—tapping her on the arm. A gray-haired grandmother held a rough and tumble toddler by his hand, and two teenage girls rubbed shoulders. All were silent as the haunting notes of *Butterfield's Lullaby* ascended into the air—a single bugler played them with meticulous precision—*Day is Done*. I felt each note and wept openly.

After the family reunion, it was all downhill—by July 12, 2004, Ted was back in the hospital. Symptoms of graft versus host plagued him, and signs that his cancer may be returning required constant monitoring. The doctors tried a little of everything, as if concocting a witches' brew, but they could not materialize a magic antidote. Even though my blood was now his blood, nothing seemed to matter. Teddy was slipping away. Again, on July 21st, I had that nagging sense of urgency that I needed to see my brother. My sister Dolly had it, too. It was 8:00 in the evening when we left for MGH.

With my adopted mantra running through my head, "It is better to look good than to feel good," I donned my red, sleeveless, knit sweater and neatly outlined my eyes in black eyeliner. I curled my lashes in upward fashion with matching mascara. I made sure my hair was presentable and my jeans fit properly. My sandals were comfortable and just okay. When Dolly and I walked into his room, Teddy tried to lift his head from his pillow. The purple, blue, and yellow bruise covering the left side of his face made me want to wince, but I tried to ignore it. He sustained it from a fall when he went walking alone in the middle of the night. Now, he was bruised on the outside as well as the inside. What else would he have to endure? He smiled; and in his soft voice he said, "You look great. Red looks great on you...kinda lookin' sexy." It was worth the extra effort. Then, feeling guilty that he was giving me too much attention, he looked at Dolly, "You look great, too." Dolly was glad she came.

I squeezed by the IV pole and bent to give him a kiss. He whispered in my ear, "You're great." It was not, "I love you" this time; but, "You're great." A shiver ran down my spine—I understood where he was coming from and squeezed my eyes shut. I hugged him hard, whispering back, "You are, too."

He pulled himself up to a sitting position and filled us in on his recent conversation with his doctor, "Dr. McKnight was just in here and he is thinking about putting some of my frozen cells back in me."

"Why would he want to do that?"

"They're wondering if it might counteract some of my graft versus host symptoms."

"Wow, Ted, that sounds so bizarre. First they wanted you to be totally converted to my cells and now they want to go backwards."

"They're just wondering if that might help."

"How do you feel about that?"

He was still holding the twisted rope of hope that something could be done, "I'm not sure, but I might let them do it."

I didn't have an answer. I didn't know what to think. It sounded crazy to me, "I guess you have to do what you feel is right for you."

He shrugged it off and turned to Dolly, "So, have you been runnin' lately?"

Dolly wasn't sure she should talk about her running because it was something he liked to do and couldn't. We had talked about that on the way to Boston. She flashed me a funny look and gave him a short reply, "I've been runnin' some, but not as much as when I was trainin' for the marathon."

"What's your problem, girl? You have to get out there."

"I know, Ted, I will."

When he started getting sleepy we told him to get some rest and tiptoed out of his room. Reaching the nurses' station, I saw Dr. McKnight behind the counter. I motioned Dolly to stop so that I could speak with him. I was able to get his attention and he came closer behind the desk.

"Ted just told us you are thinking about giving him back some of his frozen stem cells."

"It's something we are considering. We're thinking it might help with the graft versus host symptoms. It would be up to Ted."

"Some of us that have been visiting aren't sure what we should be saying to him. I want to be able to be open with him, but it's hard to know what to say."

"Ted knows that he is dying. We've talked about it. It's okay to talk with him. He has his Living Will and the chaplain has visited. Ted's a remarkable guy."

I felt comfortable with Dr. McKnight and his manner reassured me that I could ask him my questions. It was nearing 11:00 PM and he was still working. He didn't brush me aside. I had one last question.

"I think I know the answer but I just have to ask. Ted's problems now don't have anything to do with my cells being bad?" I needed confirmation.

Dr. McKnight smiled and he looked me in the eyes, "No. It doesn't."

Tears were streaming down Dolly's cheeks as she listened to our conversation. When Dr. McKnight went back to his charts she said to me, "I haven't told Teddy how much I love him."

I felt strongly for her, "You can go back in his room and visit with him alone. You haven't had that chance, and now you do. Go ahead, I will wait out here. You need to do this."

I watched her walk slowly back to his room. She had her moment alone. Dolly, being the youngest, did not have the same experiences with Teddy that I did. I was two years younger than him, she was ten. She has her own memories. We grew up in the same family, but not at the same time. Dolly was afraid she didn't really know Ted, and that's what she wanted to unload.

In the privacy of Ted's hospital room she said it out loud, "I don't feel like I really know you."

He grinned at her and raised his right eyebrow, "Yeah, ya do." It was all she needed to hear.

A second set of taps echoed the first. Far, far away from the bewitched mourners, *Butterfield's Lullaby* played again. Over the hillocks and beyond the myriad of gray gravestones, a second bugler stood alone in the woods—somewhere near Grampa Bodwell's memorial. Heard, but not seen, this marching band member made an impression—one note at a time. Morning's light flickered on the tips of green leaves and brightened pink geraniums. A soft breeze carried the tune. Day… I closed my eyes. Is… I listened intently. Done…I cried some more. I knew he was in the woods, he had to be, his bugle sounded so crisp and so clear. Yet, I could not see him. Like a mime behind a curtain, he was tangible, but not visible. Each time he exhaled, I felt a weight dragged across the currents of air, and it hovered above the dead. Lights out. Eyes shut, enveloped by this melody, I stood in darkness. In a trance, I wanted it to last longer than it did.

"Ted is breathing hard and they are going to give him a shot of morphine. You may want to come earlier than you thought."

How difficult it must have been for Corey to make this call. He was calling his grandparents from MGH to let them know that his dad was dying. If his grandmother wanted to see her son alive, she would need to leave in the next few hours. Dad had already decided he would not make the drive and I didn't want to go either. It was right for the nurse, the mom, and the social worker to be the ones to go. It wasn't a time for all of us.

Within the next hour, Mom, Becky, and my niece Laurie were on their way to Boston. When they arrived, it was Dorothy who greeted them at Ted's door, "Ted died about a half an hour ago. The chaplain is with Brenda, Corey, and Kevin. They were all with him when he died. I'm so sorry."

Coming out of my trance, I wiped my eyes as Becky strolled over.

"I heard you were having a cook-out. What time did you want people to come?"

"I told everyone to come around noon time, but Debbie can't make it until 1:00."

"Who's comin'?"

"Ronnie and Jane, Dad and Mom, Debbie, Emily and maybe Joey, all said they could make it. Of course, Jason and Derek will be there, and Alex. I think Dolly and Scott are coming, too. I'm not sure about Myles."

"You're so good to do this. Would you like me to bring a dessert and my macaroni salad?"

"Sure. That would be good."

I moved against the crowd, glancing at the stones—Ira Blake and his wife Dorothy Sanborn, and the pink peony bush. People were walking toward the street as I was walking to the back of the cemetery. For a small town, they had just put on one of the most meaningful ceremonies I had ever witnessed. I wanted to remember the details. There are details worth recording. Retrieving my bike, I thought about the bodies beneath me, long since laid to rest. What loves had they shared? What lives had they led? What secrets were buried with them? I wondered, is death nothing at all? I swung my leg over the center bar and pushed down on the pedal, settling into the padded seat of my bike. I dodged the bigger rocks in the dirt path, and swerved to miss the ditches.

When my cell phone rang I knew what to expect. Becky called from the hospital to tell me what I already suspected, "Teddy died around 3:30. Brenda, Corey, and Kevin were with him when he died. We're going to help Brenda gather his things and we'll be home later. I'll call Muffy and Dolly. Laurie will call Debbie. You can let Jimmy and Dad know."

Standing on my front porch, breathing in the scent of freshly mown grass, I held the phone to my good, right ear. (It's my left one that fills with wax.) I heard everything Becky said and I had seen enough. It was impossible to know if Ted was aware that Skippy, Jimmy and I were there the day before. I saw him in pain. He had grimaced when he changed positions. He was non-responsive. The doctors were talking about putting in a catheter. He couldn't pee on his own—standing or sitting. I didn't want him to be invaded anymore. After seeing him in that condition I prayed Ted would die. It was because I loved him so much. I loved him so much it hurt. I sighed with relief, "I'm so glad he doesn't have to suffer any longer."

A car door slammed shut as I glanced at Kensington Grange No 173 and turned right onto Trundle Bed Road. A new development of mansion-like homes had sprung up in Grampa Bodwell's farming neighborhood. (I wondered what he would have thought of them.) I stood up and peddled harder on the hill approaching the back side of the farm. Fortunately, the stately brick home on the left looked much the same as it did the day Grampa moved into town. Leveling off, and sitting back down again, I reached the top of the hill. Free to do as I pleased, I gripped my handle bars and tucked my knees in close to my bike. (Pat told me it would help me to go faster.) I bent over (to break the wind) and flew down the huge hill—gliding past the farm, and past the cow barns before I drifted to a stop. Not satisfied, I turned my bike around and peddled back to the barn. The red, faded barn boards were cracked and peeling. I pulled in close to the open barn doors and said hello to a couple of strangers standing outside the milk room. A woman, wearing a blue print dress, had medium-length brown hair and a friendly smile. She was leaning on the handle of her child's stroller. The brown, curly-haired child was content to sit there.

As I dismounted my bike and headed inside the barn, I tried to reassure the woman, "I'm not just a stranger, I'm Hal's cousin."

She laughed, "So, what cousin are you? Are you here for Harry's birthday party?"

"No. That's just for the aunts and uncles, and brothers and sisters."

"Do you live around here?"

"Yes. I live in East Kingston."

"Oh. I know Hal has a lot of family."

"Yeah. Don't even try to figure us out."

I chuckled under my breath as I walked across the strewn hay, and under the supporting beam midway through the barn. There were no cows secured in their yolks making chewing noises. I reached my hand up and easily touched the beam. The floor of the barn was not ten feet from the second floor. Guess I thought it was a lot higher than it was. I would make a note of that.

Climbing the dusty aluminum ladder, I tried not to get too dirty. Didn't there used to be a wooden ladder attached to the side of the stalls? Reaching the top, I planted my feet on the wooden surface, covered in yellow straw. I walked to the middle and looked across the barn—the distance from where I was standing and the opening in the doors was a short flight—but, without steady hands and strong arms it would hurt to fall to the ground. It was still intimidating and I would think twice before grabbing a rope and swinging into the air. I got closer to the edge to get my bearings. Ted would have been through the door and back before he gave it a second thought. I stole a last look at the cobwebs strung from rafter to rafter and at the slanted grain chute that reached up through a hole in the roof. Like my daughter would say, "It was time to move on."

I pushed "End" on my cell phone and set it on our log table. I walked across the tarred path to next door, down the curved, stone walk, past the horseshoe pits, and into Dad's back yard. Late July's heat was drying the weathered wicker basket of pink and red impatiens. The carved, wooden statue—a man and a woman embracing—stood motionless beside the well. It was Mom and Dad's fiftieth wedding anniversary gift. A bronze-colored hen clucked noisily as I drew closer to the chicken coop and her flock chimed in. Loose feathers scattered the pen. Dad, dressed in navy blue overalls and a red flannel shirt, was shingling the roof.

"Dad," I looked up to him, "you might want to come down from there."

His usual happy-go-lucky demeanor disappeared. He knew why I was there. He nodded, put down his hammer, and climbed down the ladder resting on the edge of the roof. I braced my foot against the last rung so it wouldn't shift. Calmly, head down, he waited for the news.

"Is it Teddy?"

"Becky just called. Teddy died before they got there."

He shook his head and started to cry, "Does Jimmy know?"

"Not yet. I'm going to call him next. I know he is on his way to Kelsey's soccer game. I don't want to call him while he's driving. But, I'm afraid if I wait he'll be mad. I know I have to call him now."

Wiping his eyes, he agreed, "Yeah. You better. He will want to know as soon as possible."

Smells of cow manure, cut grass, hay, and tilled earth suspended me in a time, and in a place. I peddled slowly down Stumpfield Road. I came upon the same woman that had been in the barn. She was pushing her stroller. I glided up close enough to start a conversation, "How long have you lived in Kensington?"

"About fifteen years."

"What do they say? You have to live here twenty years before you're not a newcomer? We natives are touchy about that stuff."

"I heard it was thirty."

"I'll give you twenty."

She laughed and I asked her another question, "Where did you come from?"

"I come from Massachusetts, but my husband was from around here."

"Oh. That explains it. He just had to get back to his roots."

Still smiling she commented, "I'm getting used to it. It's a good place to live."

"Where is your house?"

"It's across the pond from Hal's place."

Pushing down on my right foot, I got ready to pick up the pace. I pulled ahead of her and looked back over my shoulder. Feeling cocky I left her in my dust, "Well. Your neighbors are the best!"

Jimmy was less than prepared. As soon as my words left my lips, he hollered into the phone, "I should have been there!" I knew he would take it hard.

I tried to make him understand, "No, Jim. You've been with Ted all along. He has felt every bit of your love and concern. Don't do that to yourself. Brenda, Corey, and Kevin were with him when he died. That's how it was meant to be. You've done everything you possibly could. He knows how much you loved him. Trust me, he knows it. Please don't be so hard on yourself."

One longer downhill and I'd be pretty close to home. Looking left towards Carmen's Diner, I made sure there were no oncoming cars before pulling onto Route 108. I took my hands off the brakes and put my body in a tuck. I wanted to feel an adrenaline high. I gathered speed. I wanted to go fast. "Cruisin', not wantin' a bruisin'," I sailed by the old Dunkin Doughnuts place, an open field, and a small pond. A flock of Canadian geese were about ready to take off. I sailed by them, too. At the bottom of the hill, I coasted for as long as I could. It wasn't until I got close to another uncle's house that I had to start peddling again. It is the big yellow farm house on the left, with white trim and a tall silo. I had to stop and hold my bike for a blue mini-van before I could take a left onto Sanborn Road.

Alone, Mom walked into Ted's hospital room. It was after the immediate family had time to spend with the hospital chaplain, and after they had had their private moments with Ted. Like the dummy, Charlie McCarthy, Ted was propped up in a sitting position in his bed. His neck and shoulder muscles were life-less, and his head slumped against his pillow—tipping his all-too-familiar yellow, baseball cap to the left. The striking purple, blue, and yellow bruise escaped under his hat and spread down his left cheek. The injury was insulting. A loose, sterile johnny covered portions of his deflated chest. His bloated belly rose under a layer of white sheets. His skin was marked by increased levels of bilirubin. His feet were swollen. He came into this world yellow, and he would leave this world yellow. Ted's eyes were closed. Unable to keep his jaw shut, his mouth hung open, as if ready for someone to pull the strings. A small, cuddly, teddy bear, with an Olympic medal draped around its neck, was tenderly placed in the crook of his left arm. It was a gift from Brenda and traveled with him from Dartmouth Hitchcock to MGH. The ever-present IV pole was finally gone and Mom slipped easily to the side of his bed. Mom leaned over, reached around his cap, and kissed him on his cheek, "I love you. May you be at peace."

Mom walked away from his bed and across to the other side of the room. Lingering, she measured the meaning while she gazed out his tall, glass window with a view of the Charles River. She took one last look around his room before departing. A single, plain sheet of paper with a few quickly scrawled letters was dangling against the metal, silver bed railing. Laurie had written the words and taped it there. She had visited her uncle a few days before and when she left that evening, Ted had fallen asleep. Laurie was afraid that he would wake up and find her gone without having said good-bye. She wanted to leave him a sign: WE LOVE YOU, TED. LOVE, THE CLARK CLAN.

Dark, threatening clouds drifted across the sky, as I rode across the railroad tracks—slowly they had begun to appear. Perhaps it was going to rain after all. I better get home before it does. I peddled past "U.F.O field" (curious U.F.O enthusiasts used to park their cars by the side of the road and hope for a sighting); past "parking pull-out" where teenagers used to park where the new dusty blue house now stands; and past the white cape with rocking chairs on the front porch where Dad sold his last baby lamb. It was Memorial Day and all was quiet in my neighborhood. My neighbors were still inside. I turned into my driveway and drifted down the small slope. I put on my brakes, climbed off, and walked my bike to the tan, shingled shed.

Putting my kickstand down next to the potting soil, I glanced at the baby blue, plastic bucket of garden tools. Green flowered, garden gloves were caked with mud, and dirt was dried on the yellow spade. Maybe, I'll get a chance to do some planting. I pulled the bottom half of my shirt up, bent my head down, and made a swipe from my forehead to my chin. I'll have to throw this shirt in the wash. My LL Bean raincoat wasn't necessary but I made sure I didn't leave it in the shed. I walked across the brick path and up the red granite front step. Reaching for the black handle, I could hear Boris crying. He was waiting for me behind the door. I scooped him up before he could get away. Vigorously, I gave him a well-deserved scrubbing—with the fur and against it—and scratched his belly. I walked across the kitchen and started water boiling for my macaroni salad. In the den, I turned on my computer. Now, I could begin my last chapter.

THE END